Cancer Care By Medical Providers:

Insights and Reflections

Dr. Richard Farmer

Cancer Care By Medical Providers: Insights and Reflections
ISBN 979-8-9873623-4-1 Softbound
ISBN 979-8-9873623-5-8 Hardbound

Request for information should be addressed to:
Curry Brothers Marketing and Publishing Group
P.O. Box 247 Haymarket, VA 20168

Executive Editing by Candace Curry-Williams
Cover Design and Graphics by Vibranium Media Group
Manuscript Formatting Vibranium Media Group

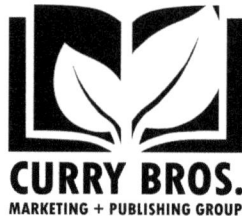

CURRY BROS.
MARKETING + PUBLISHING GROUP

Cancer Care By Medical Providers:

Insights and Reflections

Dr. Richard Farmer

Table of Contents

Cancer Care By Medical Providers: Insights and Reflections

Meet the Authors

In addition to the senior authors Richard E. Farmer and Bonnie C. Farmer, the other authors, with a brief summary of their professional experiences follows.

Richard E. Farmer, PhD

Richard E. Farmer is the former President of the Maine College of Health Professions having retired due to his health status with Multiple Myeloma Cancer. Dr. Farmer possesses an undergraduate degree from Saint Anselm College, a graduate degree from the University of New Haven, and a Doctor of Education degree from Boston University. He is a psychologist, faculty member, and academic administrator. His psychological practice has focused on stress management issues for police, first responders, and government employees. His former presidencies were at Sanford-Brown College and McIntosh College. He held senior administrative positions at Ohio Dominican University, Saint Leo University and Providence College. He also held tenured full professorships at the University of New Haven, Sacred Heart University, and Cape Cod Community College. Dr. Farmer is the author of three books, two book chapters, ten refereed journal articles, numerous newspaper articles and professional monographs, and a multitude of research papers presented at professional societies.

Bonnie C. Farmer, PhD

Dr. Bonnie Farmer is a former tenured Associate Professor of Nursing with an emphasis in Gerontological Nursing and Leadership at the University of Southern Maine. Prior to this, she was a tenured Nursing faculty member at Southern Connecticut State University. She possesses undergraduate degrees in Nursing from Northeastern University and Saint Anselm College, a Master of Public Administration and Health Care Management from the University of New Haven and a Ph.D. in Nursing from the University of Rhode Island. In addition, she holds a Certificate in Geriatric Education from the University of Connecticut and an Executive Certificate in Health Policy and Management from the Harvard University School of Public Health. She retired in spring 2014 from teaching to pursue an independent project with colleagues that would advance gerontological nursing knowledge of the older adult within nursing education and ultimately clinical practice. In late fall 2014 she became and remains a full-time caregiver to her spouse diagnosed with Multiple Myeloma Cancer. In early 2015 she was diagnosed with invasive ductal breast cancer and was successfully treated with surgery, radiation, and chemotherapy. Her perspectives written in these pages come from three different viewpoints: Her own Breast Cancer diagnosis and successful treatment, her caregiving to her spouse, and her academic and experiential background as a Nurse.

Stacey Akeley, B.S.N., R.N., CHPH

Stacey Akeley holds a Bachelor of Science degree in Nursing from Saint Joseph's College in Standish, Maine and is a Certified Hospice and Palliative Care Nurse. Her over 30-year career has spanned several areas of nursing including critical care, home health, and chronic disease care management. In all these settings and roles, she has facilitated serious illness and end of life conversations for patients and families while supporting their wishes and goals of care along the health continuum. She is currently the manager of Gosnell Memorial Hospice House at Hospice of Southern Maine where she leads and supports the employees working at Gosnell House with the same loving compassion, she has shown her patients over the years.
Lawrence Berk

Lawrence Berk, PhD

Dr. Lawrence Berk comes from a medical family, with four generations of physicians. He originally planned to go into the History and Philosophy of Science, but he was warned by the schools there were no jobs for PhD's in this field. Believing them, he instead got a PhD in physical chemistry from Yale University, studying the high field conductivity of dilute aqueous solutions. While working as a research industrial chemist he realized he should be a doctor. He quit working and went to the University of Pittsburgh School of Medicine, planning to be an ophthalmologist. He found he did not like surgery and looked around for other options. Radiation Oncology's technical and clinical aspects appealed to him, and he went on to complete his residency at the University of Pennsylvania. Throughout the process he kept up his interest in the history and philosophy of medicine. As part of this interest, he studied alternative forms of medicine, such as Traditional Chinese Medicine. He has an online degree from China in traditional Chinese medicine, allowing him to fix his computer with acupuncture. His philosophic bent led him to focus his research interests on symptom management and palliative care. He ran several national trials on the treatment of cancer symptoms. He also became board-certified in Hospice and Palliative Care. Philosophically he is a neo-Spinoza. Outside of medicine and philosophy, he also is in his 30th year and 40th iteration of trying to write the great American novel.

Elliot Cazes, M.D.

Dr. Elliot Cazes was born and raised in New Jersey. His undergraduate education was at the University of Connecticut, where he received a B.S. with Honors in Cell Biology. He then went on to obtain his M.S. in Human Physiology at Georgetown University. His medical training occurred at the University of Maryland, where he obtained his M.D. degree and completed his residency in Ob/Gyn.

Dr. Cazes has been in private practice in Tampa, FL since 1995. He has an active interest in teaching, with appointments at several universities. His areas of special interest are contraception, menopause, endometriosis and pelvic pain, abnormal uterine bleeding, and wellness and self-improvement. He has also actively pursued public speaking on women's health issues as they relate to cancer and also has spoken on behalf of many pharmaceutical companies, laboratories and charitable organizations.

In his spare time, Dr. Cazes pursues running, walking and biking. He is an avid fan of gourmet cooking, has a food blog with a growing fan base. He is a regular chef for the Faces of Courage "cancer camp" in the Tampa Bay area and for a number of other local charities. He and his wife, Pam, have raised 4 beautiful children.

Kevin O'Kelly, M.D.

Dr. Kevin O'Kelly was born in Toronto and aspired to be a doctor at an early age. His father, a physician, had immigrated from Ireland and became a urologist after training at the University of Toronto. Kevin's mother was a pediatric nurse who met his father while attending University College Galway. Growing up in a medical family allowed Kevin to see the joy in practicing medicine and inspired him to become a doctor.

In elementary school and high school Kevin struggled to be an 'A' student due to his prioritizing sports ahead of academics. Kevin and his family moved from Toronto to Columbia, SC where he attended his final year of high school. Kevin attended the University of South Carolina where he played soccer and earned his BS degree in Biology. Kevin attended medical school at St George's University, School of Medicine. He completed a general surgical residency in Brooklyn, NY, and a residency in urology at the University of South Florida which is where he met Dr. Lester Persky who was a professor emeritus at Case Western Reserve University in Cleveland, OH and Professor of Urology at the University of South Florida. Dr. Persky, along with Dr. Jorge Lockhart, trained Dr. O'Kelly to become a urologist.

Upon completion of his residency, Dr. O'Kelly entered private practice in 1993 with Florence Urological Associates. He continued his academic interests with teaching family practice residents. In 1995, Dr. O'Kelly started his own private practice at Low Country Urology Associates where he practiced solo general urology for 22 years. He performed the first robotic prostatectomy in South Carolina. Dr. O'Kelly has served as president of the Florence Medical Society, as well as president of the SC AUA. He has served on the membership committee of the S.E.S AUA. Dr. O'Kelly was previously chief of staff at Carolinas Hospital System in Florence, SC, and a board member at Carolinas Hospital System before joining the MUSC Health Marion Medical Center. Dr. O'Kelly's interests include urology and academic medicine.

Helen Ryan, M.D.

My journey to becoming an oncologist is unique. As a young girl I had always wanted to be a doctor. I loved the smell of my pediatrician's office and loved visiting there. My pediatrician was very charming, and I decided that I wanted to be a doctor. I considered doing a pre-med concentration as an undergraduate, but I loved studying literature, so I became an English major instead. After graduating from college, I took a position as a secretary for a Pediatric Hematologist in Boston. Working in that office again sparked my interest in medicine. I began taking classes at a post-baccalaureate program to satisfy the requisite pre-med courses to get into medical school. To gain more experience in the clinical realm I took a position as "Unrelated Bone Marrow Transplant Coordinator." I worked with a team of Bone Marrow Transplant physicians helping to find donors for patients who did not have family donors. It took me four years to complete my studies and I was then accepted to medical school at Tufts University in Boston. I was considered an "older" student at 27. My goal was already formed: to become an oncologist with a focus in malignant hematology. And that is what happened. After my training and completion of an internal medicine residency program, I joined an academic program for two years then moved to Maine and became a malignant hematologist within a private practice. I am currently associated with Southern Maine Health Care Biddeford Hospital.

David Persky, Ph.D., J.D.

David W. Persky is the former tenured full professor of Criminal Justice at Saint Leo University. H holds an undergraduate degree from Southern Methodist University, a master's degree in counseling from Miami University of Ohio, a Ph.D. in Higher Education from Florida State University and Juris Doctorate degree from Stetson University College of Law. Dr. Persky held a variety of administrative and academic positions at the University of South Florida and Saint Leo University. Just prior to his retirement from Saint Leo, he was diagnosed with prostate cancer. He successfully completed radiation therapy and is currently in remission.

David has been highly active in a variety of community service and honor's organizations. He has been a member, president, and district governor for Civitan International. He has served as a volunteer for the Special Olympics, a member of the greater Tampa Chamber of Commerce and a national executive member and International President for the Kappa Sigma Fraternity. He has been highly active in a number of honor societies including the Alpha Phi Sigma Criminal Justice Honor Society, Who's Who in the South and Southwest, and the Omicron Delta Kappa National Leadership Honor Society. Finally, Dr. Persky received great honors for his work at a number of Florida Universities on the creation and development of a student alcohol abuse program called "My Brother's Keeper".

Introduction to Medical Providers Insight Journey:
Lessons Learned

This book is the result of the experiences of providers as they have coped with being a caregiver to a cancer patient, commonly a spouse or other family member. There are five common themes or topics that each author has written. These themes have been developed by Richard E. Farmer as a result of his experience coping with his cancer diagnosis and the effect that this has had upon his life. He was diagnosed with Multiple Myeloma Cancer in the Fall of 2014. While there is at present no known cure for this cancer, Richard is in a close state of remission due to the successful treatment of chemotherapy. The themes that are presented here are reflections on personal experiences with cancer, essays, vignettes, and short stories designed to illustrate the theme. These have been developed by Richard fully based on his own experiences as a cancer patient learning to live a new and different life based upon his diagnosis.

It is vitally important for us to use the stress-behavior process to best understand what is going on with both the cancer patient and ourselves as caregivers. By knowing what is happening with both, we are in a better position to develop more healthy or less destructive behaviors. The idea here is that the more we know about the patient and ourselves, the better off we are as we attempt to construct coping behaviors which are healthy or less destructive to both the patient and the caregiver.

Book Themes

Each individual author is asked to write about their experiences with patients or themselves within the stated context of various themes. The themes that are presented here are Being a Cancer Patient, Obtaining Support, Hope, Saying Goodbye, and Living a Meaningful Life. A final theme, which is called Lessons Learned, will synthesize the five experiences as briefly described by the author's themselves and summarized by the last author, David W. Persky..

Being a Cancer Patient

This section will provide an overview of the cancer journey starting at the pre-diagnosis stage and ending at the conclusion of treatment and/or chemotherapy. This could focus briefly on how started, diagnosed; followed by including your feelings, attitudes, and so forth associated with this new status of life.

Obtaining Support

Reflections in this section might would include your views, attitudes, needs for support. A description of what support looks like to you and how it feels
when addressing how we can call on others to help us coping with our cancer. Can our support be identified when experienced? This could involve how we have reached out or not to caregivers, co-workers, fellow patients, and providers to help us better develop an understanding of our new status as a cancer patient from a healthful point of view. Does the meaning of support change over time and how? A cancer patient who has lived with uncurable cancer for six years could likely experience a change in how support is viewed. An interesting reflection might be how has support changed throughout the course of treatments, setbacks, decline, and recovery from acute medical-cancer events. And the concept of support also raises the issue of how we can reciprocate to the other members of our support group.

Hope

Hope is a critical attitude for the maintenance of positive mental health in all people and is especially critically important for the cancer patient. Possessing hope gives us the ability to purposely direct our lives in a positive direction. And hope helps us to produce a balance between living in the present and some living directed toward the future. Reflections on hope might include, for example, what do you hope for? Do the goals of your hope change over time with disease management and or disease progression? How do you as a cancer patient nurture the hope within you or from others?

Saying Goodbye

For most of us, our inner circle of "loved ones" could include spouses, life partners, children and grandchildren, parents and siblings, and close friends. It is with these individuals that we must face one of the most emotionally difficult tasks with saying goodbye. Saying goodbye is not necessarily restricted to the death bed with few moments to spare. For example, while medications can stop being effective, an infection can become critical. Or, if the average life span for a given diagnosis is three to five years, the cancer patient in year one, five years might be all one hears and sounds "pretty good". At year seven for that same patient, the same words can ring like a death knoll.

Another example of reflections by the cancer patient could include what are the words that we use to communicate that we will sooner or later go away and die – meaning being at age 58 years with a five-year life span average might imply that one does not see an infant grandchild graduate from high school, a beloved niece gets married, or a dear friend realizes her dream of becoming an accomplished musician. The challenges of saying goodbye can or cannot evoke powerful reactions and responses for both the cancer patient and the recipient of the message. Emotional preparation for the cancer patients and their "inner circles" can be essential for such difficult conversations.

Living a Meaningful Life
Living a meaningful life is important for all of us and is especially important for cancer patients. As all cancer patients know, the disease will quickly destroy meaning in one's life as we attempt to cope with an all-encompassing disease. Understanding this process is vitally important for the successful treatment of the disease. We need to come to terms with the fact that cancer has changed much about who we are; it robs the prior meaning we had about who and what we are, at least to some measure. Bearing this in mind, we have the knowledge and ability to reach within ourselves and recreate who and what we once were. Recognizing that meaningfulness is the cornerstone upon which we re-build our lives post diagnosis is the very first step in this process.

Epilogue - Lessons Learned
This section provides a summary of the various perspectives on the provision of medical care to cancer patients. As such, it is the intention of this Epilogue to summarize the various insights provided by the authors.

The Role of
Medical Providers and Cancer

By
Richard E. Farmer

To start the conversation about the effects of cancer upon the Oncologists, Palliative Care Specialists, Nurses, and a plethora of other cancer Support Staff, a poem/prayer seems to be necessary for setting the right tone for the pages which are presented. The following "mantra" was developed by Dr. Bonnie C. Farmer in 2015 and is modelled after the work of Jack Kornfield's Meditation on Loving Kindness (https://jackkornfield.com/meditation-loving kindness/. So, this is written by Bonnie Cashin Farmer (2015)
My Loving Kindness Mantra
Please say or repeat….

May you be well
May you be happy
May you have peace
May you be free
May you not suffer
May you be loved
May God grant you mercy and divine intervention

Follow with inserting names of…...

Yourself
Your Spouse
Your Family

Then……

Others, perhaps someone you know or know of who appears to need help, extra blessings, or caring thoughts

Some neutral person or stranger, someone who slammed a door in your face, or inappropriately pulled out of an intersection and almost hit your car while paying no attention Lastly, someone that you know or know of whom you dislike a little or a lot, someone who has wronged you, someone whose very name repels you.

Practicing on a regular basis, Loving Kindness has the power to open your heart and reinforce the good in the world. Please keep in mind that there is no right way to practice, just do whatever manner of practice that meets your needs.

The Relationship of Medicine and the Cancer Patient

Serving as a medical provider to a cancer patient can significantly help determine the quality of life for the patient and to some extent for the caretaker. And this view theoretically orients the medical provider who determines the diagnoses, provides treatment care, medication management, and outcome support. This book will focus on medical providers who become the principal source of care to the cancer patient. Further, this book will take a variety of perspectives on medical practices to cancer patients that are representative of the vast array of practices within the United States.

Medical providers serve as a uniquely important and powerful member of the cancer triad: the patient, the caregiver, and the medical provider. And it is the medical provider that can and does act as a go between the patient and myriad of others including pharmacists, physical therapists, caregivers, and others who constitute the care team for the cancer patient. Ultimately, it is the medical provider who oversees and supervises the work of the treatment plan.

Not only do the oncology physicians, palliative care physicians, nurses, medical aids, and others who, as a collective, but act as the medical team by also helping to ensure that medical orders are carried out, especially those that include medications and testing appointments. These can and are sometimes complicated and cover a vast array of actions, activities, and needs for communication between all parties involved in the patient's care.

The role of the provider is remarkably complicated. From being available to the patients for medical appointments and testing situations, to even helping the patient maintain their membership in the community in which they live. The provider also helps to oversees the nutritional aspects of the patient's diet as well as assisting in helping the patient to maintain their physical well-being and external exercise programs as appropriate, Finally, the provider seeks to assure that the patient receives the best of interactions from all who connect with the patient thus assuming a 'third ear' role on behalf of the patient.

This book will follow the insight of several individual medical providers. As such, it will follow the real experience of these individuals who have been responsible for the treatment of an individual diagnosed with cancer. In so doing, each individual author will describe their own personal reactions, thoughts, perceptions, viewpoints, attitudes, and beliefs specifically addressing the role of providing care to cancer patients. This provides the foundation for telling the real-life content as one's experience as a medical provider to cancer patients.

Against this backdrop, it is important to point out that at least three lives are changed with a diagnosis of cancer. When cancer strikes, 3 people are part of this event and depending upon the role, could potentially have their lives changed forever. The cancer patient and the caregiver will have their lives impacted, and the medical professional have their practices impacted to a lesser or larger extent. It is clear at the theoretical level that we are not the same people as we once were prior to the diagnosis of cancer. When that fateful meeting or telephone call when those terrifying words are spoken, our lives and professional practices are forever changed and/or analyzed for effectiveness. We will no longer be the same individual – patient, caregiver, and medical professional - that we were prior to hearing the words.

Patients are no longer the same as when they hear those words spoken by the medical provider or read the medical report regarding our chemistry and status, we eventually come to the conclusion that we are different than just prior. The patient is commonly overwhelmed with the idea that they can no longer do many or even most of the things that they have done in the immediate past. They wonder of they will die as a result of hearing those words and trying to comprehend their meaning. The medical provider realizes that their lives have changed at the utterance of the words because they will be placed in a role for which their patient has no preparation. And while they may deeply care for the patient, their lives have theoretically changed knowing that it will now bear the responsibility to care for the patient, perhaps for the rest of the patient's life. And too, there is a recognition that the physician and members of the medical team have yet another patient to care for, possibly ultimately even holding their hand as the patient closes their eyes for the very last time.

Depending upon the understanding of the medical provider, there are many aspects to understanding their role with respect that cancer plays in the patients being. Newly diagnosed people are now different than they were before in the sense that they are now cancer patients. And coping with these differences requires us to embrace the disease on a comprehensive basis. The role of the medical provider is to help the patient cope with these differences and learn to adopt them as part of their sheer existence. This is a fundamental part of assuming the providers role. Thus, the medical professional's role is to assist the patient with understanding of their cancer disease, teach or otherwise help the individual to both seek out and accept support from others.

One aspect of the role is to provide support to the patient and to seek out others to assist in the process of providing support. Accepting support on the part of the patient is often a difficult process. Patients must be helped to understand the very need that they may have with respect to support. In this regard, the medical provider must understand and appreciate the dynamics of support so that they can communicate to the patient the real value in surrounding themselves with others who are physically and emotionally present to the patient. These are individuals who can provide those important and critical tasks at the behest of the provider.

And from the provider's perspective it is important that they seek out others who can provide support-like activities to the patient under your supervision.

Maintaining hope on the part of both the provider, the patient and others is yet another vital process in the care of the patient with cancer. The presence of hope in the relationship between the patient and the provider is vital for successful coping on the part of the patient. With the successful work of the provider, the patient comes to realize that their life can be one of satisfaction and even joy dependent upon the actions of others. In this regard, the role of the provider is to help in the process of moving the patient in a direction that fosters positivity versus negativity.

The medical provider can help guide the patient in the positive direction through discussion and activities that demonstrate a positive value. And it is important to point out that this "positive direction" under medical supervision creates an understanding on the part of the patient that all parts of the experiences can have a positive and helpful element to it. It is the responsibility of the medical staff to point out and constantly emphasize that while it is cloudy outside, the sun is still shining.

Medical providers are vitally important to the patient if and when it becomes apparent that the patient will succumb to their cancer disease. While largely an unlikely event statistically speaking, the greatest fear of the patient is that their cancer will metastasize and consume their life. This is the very most difficult aspect of the role of the provider. And while it is impossibly difficult, it is nonetheless that time in the life of the relationship between the provider and the patient in which the provider can have a monumental effect upon the remaining days or months that the patient has to live. Helping the patient to say goodbye to members of their inner circle others – loved ones, family members, spouses, children, and acquaintances such as clergy, neighbors and known community members are critical to undertake. These goodbyes are difficult beyond imagination and the role of the medical provider is central to its happening as in many instances; it is the provider who can help to organize the process by providing emotional preparation to all the inner circle members and others who will participate.

Importantly, it is the medical provider that helps the patient to live a meaningful life, no matter how long it may be. As all cancer patients know, the disease can quickly destroy meaning in one's life. Understanding this process is vitally important for the successful treatment of the disease. The role is to assist others who need to come to terms with the fact that cancer has altered much of who we all are; it robs the prior meaning about who and what we are at least to some measure. Bearing this in mind, patients usually have the knowledge and ability to reach within themselves. And with the assistance of the direct help from the medical provider, patients are typically able to recreate who they once were. Providers are typically immensely helpful in recognizing that meaningfulness is the cornerstone upon which patients re-build their lives thus yielding the beginnings of a post-diagnosis life.

Medical providers serve as a uniquely important and powerful member of the cancer triad: the patient, the caregiver, and the medical provider. And it is the medical provider that can and does act as a go between the patient and myriad of others including pharmacists, physical therapists, caregivers, and others who constitute the care team for the cancer patient. Ultimately, it is the medical provider who oversees and supervises the work of the treatment plan.

Not only does the oncology physicians, palliative care physicians, nurses, medical aids, and others who, as a collective act as the medical team by helping to ensure that medical orders are carried out, especially those that include medications and testing appointments. These can and are sometimes complicated and cover a vast array of actions, activities, and needs for communication between all parties involved in the patient's care.

The role of the provider is remarkably complicated. From being available to the patients for medical appointments and testing situations, to even helping the patient maintain their membership in the community in which they live. The provider also helps to oversees the nutritional aspects of the patient's diet as well as assisting in helping the patient to maintain their physical well-being and external exercise programs as appropriate, Finally, the provider seeks to assure that the patient receives the best of interactions from all who connect with the patient thus assuming a 'third ear' role on behalf of the patient.

Finally, it is the medical provider that helps the patient to live a meaningful life, no matter how long it may be. As all cancer patients know, the disease can quickly destroy meaning in one's life. Understanding this process is vitally important for the successful treatment of the disease. The role is to assist others who need to come to terms with the fact that cancer has altered much of who we all are; it robs the prior meaning about who and what we are at least to some measure. Bearing this in mind, patients usually have the knowledge and ability to reach within themselves. And with the assistance of the direct help from the medical provider, patients are typically able to recreate who they once were. Providers are typically immensely helpful in recognizing that meaningfulness is the cornerstone upon which patients re-build their lives thus yielding the beginnings of a post-diagnosis life.

The Art and Science of Medical Providing: Caring

There is little doubt that Medical Providing is both an art and a science. Daily, they provide services to their cancer patients on what must be seen as a 24-hour basis. This requires that the new practitioner rapidly acquire the skills necessary to provide general medical care, drug distribution, food, and other forms of nutrition, plus other general care as needed.

It would seem that medical providing involves addressing the physical, psychological, and emotional elements which are at the heart of medical practice. These then become the foundation and definition of what we know as Cancer Medicine. In the end, it is the idea of caring for each other that provides the very basis of the care provided to cancer patients. We provide the care that we do because we care for and are committed to proper medical care for the patient. And, with a kind of caring and compassion at hand, we are able to understand the individual with cancer which allows us to provide for that person. And true compassion is nothing more than a heartfelt form of proper medical practice and a type of caring for the other person.

Caring is often associated with the concept of intimacy. For most, intimate knowledge of the other often produces change in ourselves. This change in effect puts us in an emotional "cage". This experience contains both positive and negative thoughts and ideas. The cage creates positivity and negativity in our thinking and behavior. Curiously, positivity seems to be on a type of emotional timer which has both a turn on and turn off emotional component while negativity has no timer in the cage. It is clearly up to us to turn the negativity off so that we are not locked into a set of thoughts and ideas that have difficulties or problems associated with it. In the very end, it is singularly up to us to take control of these thoughts and feelings that are fundamentally negative. And this process of control of thoughts is also known as coping.

So, where does one go from here?

First, incorporating the idea that intimacy changes over time must be recognized by all providers. And because of this recognition, there is a need for perspectives that will help us to embrace this change. There is a need for a model of thinking called the Stress Behavior Model. This helps us to integrate the Stress Behavior Model to fight negative issues such as Post Traumatic Stress Disorder (PTSD).

Second, with PTSD as a model for understanding, what happens to all of us when we are suddenly confronted with the knowledge that our loved one has contracted cancer? This suddenly terrifying situation can result in any number of reactions such as vivid flashbacks to a more relaxing and peaceful situations, intrusive thoughts or images, nightmares, intense distress at prior experiences with you and the cancer patient, and physical sensations at the mere thought of prior highly pleasant situations with you and the cancer patient.

Third, the PTSD reactions or other reactions can be best delt with by incorporating stress behavioral principles into your thinking about your loved one suddenly conflicted with cancer. The stress-behavior model was conceived as a method to understand what we do when confronted with things like PTSD behaviors. This is a process that includes recognition of the "stressors" we experience when we think about the cancer altering your relationship with the patient. This involves recognizing and identifying the "source" of the feeling, and the effects that this has upon us both physically and emotionally. Next comes the "effects" of the sources upon us both physically, emotionally, and socially. Finally, the coping behaviors that we employ to cope with the sources and their effects upon us.

Readers are encouraged to create a paper form in which on the left side of the paper you write the words in a column, source, effects, and behaviors leaving ample space in the column for the three words. These should cover the entire length of the paper. In the middle of the paper form, you provide a wide column to record you effects or feelings of what the source does to you either physically or psychologically. Finally, the remaining space on the paper is for behaviors that you engage in when you experience the source and effects. In the end, this will give you a tool that will assist you in being a better caregiver for your patient. So, you are encouraged to go ahead and experiment with the form even to having multiple pages of the form to cover a whole series of sources.

As one military scholar reported that they, the military, are trained to respond and not react. The idea here is that we need to "train" ourselves so that we can respond and not just react. The Stress-Behavior Model thinking is a great way to begin the process of training ourselves so that we can respond to the needs of the cancer patient, and not just react to their requests or your determination of their needs at a given moment. The idea here is that merely reacting to a situation will often not give us the best response to a caregiving situation. Rather, training ourselves to respond is by far a better form to being a good caregiver than by simply reacting "from the gut" to a caregiving situation.

Caring Then And Now

By
Bonnie Cashin Farmer, Ph.D. R.N.

The purpose of this article is to take a closer look at the role of caring in the provision of healthcare by medical providers. "Then" reflects my early academic work and research on understanding caring in clinical practice. "Now" reflects my understanding of caring today from a broader viewpoint resulting in reexamination of the efficacy of caring as an essential component of competent healthcare.

My presence in healthcare has been almost lifelong: beginning as a "candy striper" in a local hospital followed by a nurse's aide, a registered nurse in varying positions in hospitals, public and community health settings providing direct services, and lastly as a tenured nursing faculty member of two universities. Throughout all these professional experiences, I have remained committed to excellence in clinical practice.

Advancements in science, technology, and education combined with the changing values of individuals, organizations, and communities continue to influence and shape the current day practice of healthcare. Despite the challenges inherent in an ever-changing and shifting healthcare environment, excellence in clinical practice remains paramount to both medical providers and patients alike.

THEN

As a registered nurse and an Assistant Professor of Nursing, caring within the context of healthcare has long been a professional, research, and academic interest of mine. Several decades ago, as a nursing doctoral student, I had a course assignment requiring an in-depth theoretical analysis of any aspect of nursing of my choice. I naively decided to focus thinking on caring: a mainstay of the nursing profession of which I knew so well or so I thought. Eighty-eight pages of my course assignment later, I knew less than when I began and had many unanswered questions. That original work fueled further studies of mine, examining the meaning of caring within healthcare settings such as clinical practice, nursing homes and healthcare organizations. Caring, as a derivative of the word "care", appears to be a simple six letter word. In the beginning of medical history, care and cure were essentially one. Over time, as medicine became more scientific, providing cure without care increasingly became a distinct possibility.

My initial review of the caring literature sought to determine an acceptable definition of caring to guide my further academic and clinical research. It became increasingly clear to me that caring is something other than a set of mechanistic acts, developmental behaviors, or acquired attitudes. Although the definition of caring continued to be redefined and reworked, a basic premise underlying all assumptions regarding caring supports the essential role of caring in healthcare.

The very word "healthcare" can mistakenly imply the assumption of caring. Yet care and caring have distinctive meanings resulting in different images. These images of care and caring are not to be considered oppositional but rather different in orientation, perspectives, and outcomes. For example, medical and nursing scholars distinguish between taking care of patients which emphasizes objective, professional care, such as the medical and psychological aspects of healthcare and caring for patients as a humanistic way of interacting with patients.

A humanistic perspective of the provider and patient relationship emphasizes the provider seeing each patient beyond a cancer diagnosis: a unique and whole individual. Humanistic interaction is based upon honesty, empathy, compassion, altruism, humility, and reflective of respect and dignity for the beliefs of the patient and their families.

Caring can be considered a universal quality of human existence and human goodness extending well beyond the realm of medical care. Thus, caring becomes potentially inherent in all persons and relationships; with the medical provider and patient relationship being no exception. An essential element of caring as a way of being includes the idea of the presence of oneself, immersed in the here and now, and seeing self and others as human beings. Heightened sensitivity to being immersed in the here and now fosters the ability to hear and be heard, and to respect and be respected.

When such barriers are broken and there is less division between self and others, it is easier to see the caring nature of humankind. One who professes to know all the answers to the questions, to know what is right for the other, and to consider caring as a privilege, does not understand caring and cannot be open to experience genuine caring.

In very simplistic terms, caring is a way of being and a complete reflection of overall harmony with self and other. Further considerations of caring as a way of being, I leave such conversations and analyses of caring to philosophers, ethicists, writers, and critics.

The experience of caring for cancer patients is dependent upon any individual's particular view, understanding, and interpretation of caring: which means involving the personal meaning of the cancer experience and treatment effects. The individual interpretations of caring by medical providers, cancer patients, and their families are much like a set of fingerprints that are unique and non-replicable. Caring may be viewed as a kind of continuum within the context of degrees as opposed to a static product, action, or goal.

The question then arises "is caring more of an "art" as opposed to a science. For example, when a medical provider presents the facts and the evidence to support healthcare decision making, risks and benefits of interventions, and desired outcomes, the art becomes the provider's ability to communicate such evidence-based information in a manner that best reflects the individual needs of the patient. Combining both the art and science of caring, medical providers can form the foundation for excellence in clinical practice.

NOW

Now here I am years later: a retired tenured Associate Professor of Nursing, a cancer patient, and a caregiver for my spouse with multiple myeloma cancer for whom remission has eluded. I am once again taking a closer look at caring within the provision of present-day healthcare. My professional understanding of caring in healthcare remains ever-growing, questioning, and frequently disillusioning. My personal and family experiences of caring in healthcare reflect the full gamut of excellent and outstanding to mediocre at best and woefully unacceptable.

What then does caring mean to cancer patients and their families during these times of pandemics, staff shortages, supply shortages, rising costs, and decreased resources. Caring and care can become so overused, used interchangeably with minimum insight, diluted to meaningless, and result in unmet expectations of both medical providers and patients. Caring can neither be purchased nor quantified.

The plethora of healthcare satisfaction surveys of one's recent visit might suggest that healthcare organizations are caring, really wanting to hear from you, and desiring patient input for improvement of services. My own experiences suggest that despite the constant barrage of surveys, palpable change for the better remains elusive. Patient satisfaction does not necessarily reflect a caring experience.

Recently I realized how accustomed I have become to rushing to answer an anticipated phone call from a medical provider in fear of missing the call, talking fast, trying to guesstimate the shortest hold time of the day when returning a missed call to the medical office, and always having my schedule book readily available. Healthcare is a complicated and complex business for which human beings, like you and me, are dependent. A cancer diagnosis can plunge patients and their families into unfamiliar medical territory: far removed from the wellness checks and routine labs of the primary care physician's office, clinic, or community medical services.

Caring, within the context of oncology, the branch of medicine that specializes in the diagnosis and treatment of cancer, presents itself as a dilemma for both medical providers and patients: providing competent and compassionate care while meeting the deeply personal and individual needs of the cancer patient. Although all medical providers may have the capacity for caring, the demands and harsh realities of clinical practice can impair the caring experience for both provider and patient. Like for patients, pandemics, staff shortages, supply shortages, decreased resources, rising financial costs, and "bottom lines" can also negatively affect the quality of a provider's clinical practice. Medical providers, as the prominent figureheads of healthcare, are as compromised by contemporary healthcare inadequacies as are patients.

Yet, the one constant of any clinical practice is the medical providers themselves. The medical provider has the capacity to make a difference for the cancer patient, to the cancer patient, and with the cancer patient. Medical providers, as human beings, have the capacity to be fully present by bringing their whole selves to each patient and family encounter: breaking artificial barriers, demonstrating empathy and compassion, and bringing provider and patient together as they walk the cancer journey.

When an individual provider thinks of the "other" instead of oneself, the possibility of genuine caring arises: an essential act of caring is bringing one's whole self, however brief, to a conversation, discussion, or relationship, the possibilities of empathy and compassion are endless. I frequently offer wishes to my providers for a peaceful heart knowing that by doing their best every day, they make a difference for their patients, families, themselves, and me.

Are we as patients asking too much from our medical providers? I have often thought that an appreciation of the responsibilities of both the provider and the patient has the potential to enhance the medical provider/patient relationship. Genuine caring reflects the medical provider and the patient coming together as ordinary individuals. Caring may or may not be an individual attribute of provider nor patient.

Acknowledging the wide variation in practice styles of providers, with individual interpretation of caring by both patients and providers, fosters opportunities for establishing a good first step toward nurturing the caring experience. Providing medical care demands an embodiment of the notions of empathy and compassion. Empathy involves objective and active communication of understanding, being aware of, and actively being sensitive to another person. Compassion is more of an emotional response for wanting to alleviate the distress of another. *

My own expectations of medical care have shifted away from caring as an essential component of healthcare. I personally think of caring as a quality that I highly value yet remain committed to the greater importance of competent, timely, empathic, and compassionate medical care. The ever-changing landscape of healthcare today presents a quagmire of challenges for both providers and patients. Caring is admittedly threatened in contemporary healthcare.

Caring and competent care: patients and their families want both as do medical providers. Within this closer look of caring, competent medical care based upon respect for one another, preservation of dignity, empathy, and compassion can nurture the actualization of caring in contemporary healthcare. The desire for excellence in the clinical practice of today can be transformed beyond an ideal from then and now become a reality when shared by both medical providers and patients alike.

* In-depth dialogues of caring, compassion, and empathy within the context of healthcare is well documented in publications that are available and accessible online. Government sites, such as https://pubmed.ncbi.nlm.nih.gov/, area reliable resource

A Physician's Perspective On Caring For Cancer Patients: Treatment Plans, Providing Support, Hope, and Saying Goodbye

By
Lawrence Berk, M.D.

Many years ago, my then young daughter asked me what I do for a living. I told her I am in sales: I have 15 minutes to convince a patient that I am the appropriate person to treat him or her. An important part of my process to provide care to a patient with cancer is to efficiently use the interactions I have with the patient at the initial consultation. I am rarely an early provider in the cancer-care process, and the patient's records usually have most or all of the information that I need to discuss care with the patient. Therefore, prior to seeing the patient, I review all of the available information and prepare most of the consultation notes. This frees me to focus on the discussion part of the consultation, rather than spending time reviewing things the patient already knows. This also allows me to better understand what I need to be focusing on while I am with the patient. In the appropriate setting, I may walk into the room and state up front that the patient does not need radiation therapy, thereby relieving anxiety at the start of the consultation.

In the beginning of my consultation, I will proceed to briefly review his or her case to ensure that I correctly have all of the relevant details. Most cancers present in a somewhat typical pattern with available consensus guidelines recommending or not recommending radiation therapy. I use the guidelines, if available, as the starting point for the treatment discussion. The first decision is whether the treatment is "definitive" or "palliative." This is based on the stage of the cancer and the health of the patient. Definitive treatment is designed to cure the patient at the risk of short-term, and perhaps long-term, harm to the patient. The risk-benefit ratio of the treatment is sufficient to recommend the treatment.

Palliative treatment is not designed to cure the patient, but to offer an improvement in the quality of life of the patient. The same presentation of cancer may be treated as potentially curative for a fit 60-year-old, but as a palliative treatment for a frail 80-year-old. After deciding the goal of the

the treatment, if there is to be treatment, then the treatment itself can be designed. For definitive treatments, national guidelines may simplify this by stating what the patient should receive. If not, then the best outcomes from the literature are the usual basis for my treatment recommendation.

The final treatment plan usually focuses on combining what the data suggest are appropriate treatments with what the goals of the patient are, and how will the patient best be able to tolerate the treatment with the least short-term and long-term side effects. Again, most of this decision making is done before I step into the room. However, seeing and talking about treatment with the patient may change how I would approach this individual patient. And I will tell this to the patient, that generally I recommend this but because of these factors, this is what I recommend for you. This then leads to the informative part of the consultation. I describe what sort of tests the patient will have to prepare for treatment, what the planning and treatment are like, and the potential acute and chronic side effects. I try to inform the patient just how difficult the treatments could be, and how long the patient will likely be debilitated. I describe permanent changes that the patient can expect. After this, I review the main information of the consult with the patient to make sure the patient understood what was said. And then I will obtain formal informed consent from the patient for treatment.

For palliative treatments I must approach the consultation from a different perspective. No longer am I telling the patient what I think is the appropriate treatment. Now, the patient must direct me towards what is the appropriate treatment. An example is a patient with prostate cancer, and it has spread to the bones, bone metastases. The objective data, such as his imaging, tells me where the bone metastases are. It does not tell me how much pain the metastases are causing and how that affects the patient's life. Therefore, the start of my consultation for such a patient would be to probe if the patient has pain, where the pain is located, how bad is the pain, what other treatments are starting, and, importantly, what would the patient consider a successful treatment. Based upon a detailed discussion of needs and goals, I will develop and present a treatment plan. For palliative care, the risks have to be much less than the benefits.

Obtaining Support

I always try to make sure that the patient and the patient's support people understand what the cancer is, what the intent of the treatment is, how the patient will be treated and what the patient will experience during and after treatment. Many other physicians spend an hour or more at this initial consultation. I tend to spend less than twenty minutes. Twenty minutes is more than enough time to discuss why and how the patient will be treated. My belief is that spending an hour with the patient generally means the physician is talking to the patient, rather than with the patient.

How a patient finds support during their journey with cancer will be dependent on what level of support that the patient needs and what the patient brings to the table. Most cancers occur in people who are older and have already established spiritual goals and needs. A religious patient can seek help from their church. A non-religious, spiritual person will seek comfort in whatever teachings attracted the person to those beliefs. As a physician, especially a physician treating people with cancer, I need to take care to stay empathetic and not sympathetic. I acknowledge the fear and suffering that the patient has, but I have to minimize its emotional content for me. As part of my empathy, I talk with the patient, seek out if there is suffering, and try to find ways to help alleviate it. Often this is with medical treatment, such as pain medications or anxiety medications, but it can also be that the act of acknowledging the problems helps to lessen the suffering. I also educate as much as possible.

I often know what may be happening in the future, at least in general, and giving this information to the patient reduces their feeling of being adrift. If these are not sufficient, then other support personnel, including the social worker, the psychologist, the chaplain, are added to the treatment team. For some patients the most severe anxiety occurs at the diagnosis and start of treatment. Once treatment is under way, a regular routine set, and a probable outcome defined, the patient can slowly return towards their baseline functioning. Other patients, particularly the patients without a curative treatment, will travel a different path. New problems and needs will continue to arise that have to be addressed as they occur. My primary method of support in either case continues to be empathy and education.

Hope Perspectives

I do not emphasize a strong role for "hope" for the support of a cancer patient. I stress living in the moment and addressing the potential outcomes of cancer and treatment with clarity and facts. Hope suggests that there is some outside agency that is controlling the patient's fate, and that the outcome can somehow be manipulated. If the patient wants to seek assistance from a higher power, then I encourage the patient to go to their pastor. However, I do not get involved in this aspect of the patient's care. Rather, I continue to educate, to update, and to direct treatment. "Hope" can be used by a patient or family to avoid having to make difficult decisions and to avoid reality. A treatment that has a one in a hundred chance of having any benefit will have the same probability of effectiveness whether the patient is "hopeful" or not. And often, in my experience, it is the family looking for hope, not the patient. And this may lead the family to force the patient to get treatments to make the family feel better, rather than the patient. Therefore, I stress knowledge rather than hope. Part of a good death is the appropriate transitioning along the treatment pathway.

Saying Goodbye

Ultimately death is the only potential outcome of life. Death for myself or for others does not bother me. I agree with Epicurus, who stated that it is foolish to fear death. If you are alive, death is not present. If you are dead, you are not present. I fear dying. I do not want to suffer, and I want to die with dignity. Therefore, my approach with a dying patient is not significantly different from that of a non-dying patient. I want not only to relieve the patient's suffering, but I also want to maximize the quality of life of the patient. We all die, and therefore death is not unusual or unnecessary, it is both natural and unavoidable. I am satisfied with doing everything I can to assist with a good death.

Being a physician dedicated to providing care to cancer patients, the principles outlined here are designed to help the patient to cope with their cancer diagnosis. For a cancer treating physician, these principles represent a professional process which creates a treatment plan designed to help the individual to best understand their disease and to learn how to best cope.

Crucial Conversations: Insights From A Medical Provider

By
Elliot Cazes, M.D., F.A.C.O.G.

I finished my residency in Ob/Gyn in 1995 and entered the "real world" of medical practice, choosing to join a group Ob/Gyn practice in Tampa, FL. Prior to this, while I was still in medical school, I entertained the thought of becoming an oncologist. However, I quickly learned during my med school rotations that caring for cancer patients full-time was very stressful, too stressful for me. I found myself capable of working with cancer patients, but only if those encounters were surrounded by encounters with other types of patients. I did develop an interest in caring for cancer patients at least some of the time and I knew that if I entered the field of Ob/Gyn, I would encounter and care for cancer patients in the context of Ob/Gyn (Breast, Uterine, Ovarian, Cervical and other "female" cancers) on a regular basis. Residency afforded me many opportunities to care for female patients with cancer, and I quickly developed a strategy to approaching these newly diagnosed patients.

When I entered private practice, I was fairly comfortable in terms of organizing my thoughts and actions when it came to my interactions with cancer patients. As I ventured out into the world of healthcare, I wanted to be sure that I had the confidence to adequately address all of these patients' needs. I wanted to make sure that I was practicing up to the prevailing and highest standard of care when I formulated a management plan for a cancer patient. Questions raced through my mind such as "Am I making the right types of referrals?" "Am I covering all of the bases in terms of the multifaceted care that would be required?" "Am I involving the patient in care decisions whenever possible?;" and "Am I exhibiting a proper amount of empathy towards the patient?" When I went into private practice, I was confident that I was doing all of the above, and adequately. Medical school and residency prepared me well for my cancer patient encounters.

It is important to discuss what exactly goes through the mind of a medical provider when faced with a newly diagnosed cancer patient. First, it is important to realize that in most cases a cancer diagnosis cannot be anticipated, and it comes as a surprise, and a bad surprise at that. Initially, when faced with a new diagnosis, I want to be 100% sure that I am making the right call about the patient's condition, that I am reading the results correctly and I have read them thoroughly. There is absolutely no room for error when sharing a new cancer diagnosis with a patient. You do not get a second chance with a cancer diagnosis. Initially, I will reach out to the pathologist, laboratory or referring provider to confirm that we have the correct diagnosis. When I receive confirmation of the diagnosis, it is time to discuss that diagnosis with the patient. This is a difficult conversation, and it has never gotten easier during my career. It is impossible to predict how a particular patient will respond to the news.

Many patients will be shocked and devastated, and many will immediately become sad, depressed and scared at the same time. Some patients will be totally calm. It is always best to have a supporting family member or friend present when breaking the news to a patient, and I try to arrange for that whenever possible. I try to think of different scenarios to pursue based upon the patient's response to the news. They may respond very negatively, very neutrally or even see it as a challenge to overcome – this would require different strategies on my part, in response to the patients' reactions. It is never good to be caught without a plan, and I try to have each "next step" in my plan ready to go. As the patient's healthcare provider, I am there to provide the diagnosis to them. I am also there to map out the next several steps involved – appropriate referrals, additional testing, information gathering for their family members and/or support persons, insurance coverage, etc., and I try my best to be prepared for each possible eventuality. I am also there to be someone for them to lean on, someone whose shoulder they can cry on, an individual to whom they can sound off to, in terms of their surprise, their sadness, their disappointment, their anger at having received a cancer diagnosis. Interestingly, I have found that women tend to be much more comfortable and more expressive with their Ob/Gyn than with their other medical providers, and they are, therefore, comfortable with the notion of talking with us during such difficult times. Honestly, this can make our jobs somewhat easier at times, and this certainly applies to the situation in which we are discussing a new cancer diagnosis. Patients tend to be very trusting of what we tell them, and they tend to be very accepting of whom we refer them to.

As I approach the new cancer diagnosis, first and foremost, I want to make sure that I set my patient up for appropriate and adequate care for their cancer. I will not be the one providing this care, but I certainly will be helping to coordinate it. I will initially talk to the patient about quickly setting her up for an appointment with the type of oncologist suited to care for her type of cancer (in a majority of my patients' cases, this will be a gynecological oncologist). In these instances, I personally call the physician to arrange for the initial consultation, and then I immediately relay all relevant logistical information to my patient. I also arrange for all relevant records (biopsy results, labs, radiology results, etc.) to be sent to the providers that I am referring the patient to for their review and analysis before they see the patient.

I try my best to explain to the patient exactly what to expect at that first visit. I want to make the patient as comfortable as possible with the process as they prepare to head into the initial consultation with the oncologist. At this point, based upon the specific type of cancer, I will try to give the patient an "overview" in terms of what to expect prognosis-wise, leaving the specific details to be discussed with the oncologist. Again, as I have noted, I am not an oncologist, but my patients tend to be extremely comfortable with me, and I believe that it benefits them for us to have as broad a conversation as possible about their diagnosis, while they are in the "comfortable environment" of my office.

I also try to help them prepare at this point for conversations that they will be having with spouses, children, other family members and friends. These conversations will be difficult initially, and I want to prepare the patient for these conversations as well as I can. There will be questions that my patient will be asked, and I want them to be prepared to answer them. There will be other questions that my patient will have for their family and friends, and I want them to be prepared for the answers that they will receive in return. They will encounter many different types of responses as they break the news of the cancer diagnosis to people. I believe it is my job to help prepare them for the possible range of emotions. The patient will encounter sadness, rage, disbelief, sympathy, optimism, pessimism and sometimes even pity. They should be prepared to adequately deal with any of these reactions and I try to provide them with the tools to do just that.

As I complete the initial discussion of a new cancer diagnosis with the patient, it is foremost in my mind that I want them to leave my office with the feeling that they are well-informed about their particular diagnosis. I want them to feel that all of their pertinent questions have been answered. I want the patient to feel that they have had an opportunity to express their emotions, even if that means crying on my shoulder or pounding on the walls of my office. I want them to be comfortable with the plan moving forward and comfortable in knowing that I will be available to help them deal with any "issues" that may arise in that plan. I want them to feel comfortable that they will be seeing the best providers around; specialists that are very experienced with their diagnosis and from whom they will be receiving the best care that is out there for them. When my patient and I have finished discussing the new cancer diagnosis, it is imperative that we both feel that we have achieved a certain comfort level about the course of treatment. If not, we must step back and reflect and reformulate plans where necessary.

OBTAINING SUPPORT

Another important role of the medical provider is to offer and provide support to the newly diagnosed cancer patient – both logistical and emotional support. First, it is my role to make things "run smoothly" for my patient. I want to assist them in scheduling appointments, obtaining all diagnostic testing results and securing proper insurance coverage. I want to put the patient at ease and to be comfortable with the timing of appointments with the oncologist and other cancer specialists who will be involved with their treatment. The patient must have an organized package of information to bring to their cancer specialists. The patient must feel that the appointments are conveniently timed for both themselves and their support network, and that the appointments are located within relatively easy travel distance. I regularly assist my patients with these important details. I may need to spend a bit more time with the patient and going the extra yard but I strongly believe that everything should be well orchestrated so the patient will embark on this difficult journey with minimal anxiety and a sense of optimism. I will do whatever is necessary to help ease the patient's fears. I will support them with as many details as I can in terms of what to expect moving forward. I want them to be well prepared and I want them to have a realistic attitude towards everything that they will be going through on their cancer journey.

Perhaps even more importantly, it is my role to provide the newly diagnosed patient with as much emotional support as I possibly can. There is a wide range of emotions that the patient will express upon initially receiving the cancer diagnosis. Many will express anger – anger at being "the one" who has been diagnosed with cancer. Anger at the fact that they have been blindsided by the diagnosis and their life has been changed forever. I reassure the patient that nothing that they have done has caused them to be cursed with such a diagnosis. It is NOT their fault, and honestly, they probably could not have done anything to prevent the diagnosis. It is essential to make them understand this. It is bad luck or simple misfortune that they are experiencing this cancer diagnosis. It is likely that the patient will experience sadness or even depression. Sadness that their life is about to change drastically; that they might be facing their own mortality; that their family members might soon be parting ways with a loved one; that they might not be able to carry on daily functions of life in the same manner as previously.

I am here for them to vent. I am here to be a shoulder to cry on. I am here as a neutral party that does not have a daily presence in their life. Foremost, I am here to listen! As I always tell my medical, Physician Assistant and Nurse Practitioner students, "Your ears are your most important pieces of equipment as a provider, use them well!" I will listen for as long as the patient needs me to, and then I can add my guidance when the patient is ready to hear it.

The sadness that a patient experiences may border on or become major depression. As a provider, I am always on the lookout for this change. Many new cancer patients will need counseling or even medication to work through this emotion. I have no problem starting a patient on an antidepressant in order to deal with the diagnosis, as long as they are a willing party. I will not push medications on these patients, but if they ask about medications, I am glad to help out. I also have a low threshold for referring them to a mental health counselor. After all, this diagnosis presents a major life change, and the patient might need professional assistance in getting through this. I will also encourage my patient to lean on family members, friends, colleagues or anyone who is willing to support them, and in particular, any of those individuals who have already been through a similar cancer experience. These individuals can lend an incredible amount of necessary support to the patient.

It has been my experience that many patients will experience a fear or concern that they simply cannot get through this process both emotionally and logistically. I am here to reassure them that we will "get this done" together. I am here to steadily guide them through the lengthy process; there is no need to be fearful of not being successful. Having and maintaining a positive attitude is necessary to fight cancer. Fear and pessimism only serve to diminish the patient's likelihood of success in beating cancer, so they must remain positive. As their provider, I know that they will get through this if we work together as a team, and I constantly remind them of that. The journey will be long, and it will not be easy. There will be difficult moments and difficult days, but we can get through it if we stay focused on the goal at hand – beating cancer. Dwelling on failure will only serve to darken a patient's outlook, so I do whatever is in my power to foster an outlook that success will occur.

All of these emotions can be difficult for a patient to deal with. However, if we deal with them appropriately from the outset, the chances of a positive outcome are increased. There is no emotion that we cannot deal with. We must confront each emotion as the patient experiences them. I cannot stress how much a patient will depend on the support that their provider has to offer. Medical providers must fulfill the promise to always be there for the patient throughout this lengthy process!

SEEKING AND OBTAINING HOPE
The medical provider serves a vital role in assisting the patient in seeking and obtaining hope throughout the entire cancer battle. Receiving a cancer diagnosis often puts patients in the position of having a negative outlook from the outset and moving forward. Many patients have difficulty believing that there is hope, and that there could be a "happy ending" to their cancer journey. Some patients give up hope very early in the process and often become so bogged down in the logistics of dealing with emotions and of seeking proper and adequate care, that they overlook the importance of moving forward with a sense of hope and a positive outlook. Early on during this process, I sit down with each patient for a lengthy conversation to discuss the need to have hope and the need to remain positive. While a cancer diagnosis can be devastating for a patient to receive, it is imperative to explain to them that many patients will survive, many will go on to live very productive and happy lives once this chapter in their lives concludes. It is absolutely essential that, as a provider, I help them understand that they must believe from the outset that they will survive and will ultimately get

past the shock of a cancer diagnosis and have a happy ending. I share with them the most current, accurate statistics and prognostic data on their particular type of cancer.

The survival rate has improved for many cancers in recent years, and I make sure that each patient truly understands this. I provide them with written and online resources that they can review to remind themselves of this positive trend. I try to be honest and candid at all times, but I stress the positive and downplay the negative. I try to connect them with cancer specialists who share this same view of the importance of positivity and hope. I also connect new cancer patients with other patients who have gone through the same process and ended up doing well – having happy endings and ringing the bell to defeat cancer. "Experienced" patients are a valuable source of positive guidance for new patients. There is something special about being able to connect with another individual who has gone through the same process and come out with a positive outcome. It is also important to me that I constantly encourage my patients along the way to wake up each day with a positive outlook, rather than dwelling on the negatives of their diagnosis. Cancer is scary and cancer is truly a "bad thing" that we don't want anyone whom we care for to have to go through. But we do the patient a big favor when we remind them to be positive each and every day and to be grateful for all of the good things that they do have going on. The patient needs to realize that she is surrounded by friends, family and providers that want nothing but to see them succeed in beating their cancer diagnosis. These are people for whom the patient should be grateful. They can build off of the positive energy of these individuals each and every day that they deal with their diagnosis.

It is also very important to ensure that the patient's family members (an incredibly important source of support on a daily basis) are on board with the suggested treatment plan. It does not benefit the patient to be surrounded by family members who exude negative energy, and I will often have a discussion with family members about the need to remain positive at all times and to stress that there is, indeed, hope out there for our patient. This helps our patient to navigate the daily ups and downs that they will experience during their cancer journey. If I can help a patient to secure hope, then I can certainly help them to maintain this sense of hope. And if we can maintain hope and positivity, then all aspects of the patient's experience with cancer will be made much easier to navigate.

It is important that I help my patient obtain hope immediately after receiving the cancer diagnosis. It is equally important that I help them maintain hope throughout their time with me. I am a very strong believer in the power of positive thinking – I have seen how much better patients do when they have a positive outlook, as opposed to those who continue to feel a very negative vibe. I work very hard at constantly reminding my patients to wake up each and every day with a positive attitude. I strongly believe that it makes a difference in terms of outcomes. The medical aspects of the patient's cancer diagnosis "are what they are," but the significance of a positive attitude can never be downplayed. It is possible for a patient who has cancer to go on and live a very happy and productive life – let us never forget this!

SAYING GOODBYE

It is never easy to prepare to say goodbye to a patient who has endured the cancer journey. It is not easy for the patient. It is not easy for their family, loved ones and friends. And it is never easy as a provider. I have been in practice for over 27 years, and I still find it extremely difficult to say goodbye. But it is important to prepare everyone for this eventuality. At some point, it will become apparent that a patient is not going to recover from their cancer diagnosis, and that the end is near. This may be a gradual realization in a patient who was previously doing well with their treatment, or it can come more suddenly with an unexpected turn for the worse in the patient's health status. Either way, it is important to realize when a cancer traveler has reached this point and it is important to prepare for the events that will occur moving forward.

A patient should be prepared to "get their things in order" financially, legally and of course, emotionally. As a provider, I cannot help them get things in order, but I can and often do provide moral support and words of encouragement. I direct them to individuals who will be able to assist the patient in these matters. I can be there to listen if they need a sounding board of sorts or wish to vent. I encourage them to reach out to others who will play a key role in this process. I can help a patient compile a list of those individuals with whom they will want to speak before their passing. If I am asked, I can help them gather the right words to say and I can help to make sure that they don't overlook anyone. Each patient has a different perspective on exactly what they want to say and on how to say their goodbyes. Some patients want these conversations to be lengthy and "all inclusive," while others prefer to keep it fairly brief. Some patients find it very difficult if the conversations are drawn out and lengthy. I have offered guidance many times to help patients to determine just how much they want to say. There have been instances when I will consult with both the patient and their significant other or other family members in order to make this transition easier for the patient. This part of the process needs to be about the patient first and foremost and less about those to whom they are saying goodbye. As I always like to say, "no regrets," meaning that it is important to say goodbye and to clear the air in a manner in which the patient will move on without looking back with regrets. I clearly remember when my father passed away several years ago. We had been having some difficulties in our relationship, and so it was very important that we cleared the air prior to his saying goodbye and passing on. We did that, and to this day, I have no regrets. I share this with my patients, as it is my hope that they will do the same. I hope that they will pass on without regretting not clearing the air where necessary. As part of the process of saying goodbye, I encourage my patients to dwell on the positives and not on the negatives. I do not want them to think about the negative aspects of this horrible disease as they approach the end of their journey. It is better that they focus on the positives – the important people in their lives, the things that they have accomplished, the wonderful positive memories of all of the years of their lives. They should look back fondly on all of these and be at peace when they do eventually pass on.

Saying goodbye never gets any easier. It is a painful, difficult process that is full of a wide range of emotions, and it is important for me to be a part of this final process that my patient goes through. My goal is to make it easier and to make it as positive an experience as possible, given the circumstances.

DEVELOPING A MEANINGFUL LIFE
As a medical care provider, it is important to help a patient newly diagnosed with cancer to realize that although their time may be limited, they can still live a meaningful life. All of the steps that are outlined in this book are extremely important, yet this last one is perhaps the most important part of the cancer journey. Once a patient has gotten over the initial shock, and once they have formulated a game plan for appropriate treatment, I take time to sit down with the patient to come up with a plan as to how they will live out the rest of their life. That does not mean that they will not outlive the cancer and be a "survivor." Whether a patient ultimately dies from the cancer or goes on to live as a survivor, it is important to make the remainder of their life worthwhile. In my experience, it is essential that the patient sit back and an analyze which facets of their lives are most important. What are

their top priorities? Who are the people that they want to spend more time with? What dreams do they have that are unfulfilled? Are there things that they still want to do, places that they still want to visit? To use a cliché, this is the time for them to formulate a bucket list! Now that they have confronted a cancer diagnosis, it is time to make the most out of every remaining day and every remaining minute.

I tell my patients that despite the cancer and the difficult, horrible experience that they have gone through – life is still very much worth living. Some patients will feel stigmatized due to their cancer diagnosis, and I tell them that this is simply not something that they should be concerned with. They may feel that, now, their lives are "tainted" in some way, and again, I tell them that it is not so. They should be happy to be alive for whatever amount of time remains. They should greet each new day with happiness, excitement and gratitude. Often, a patient will feel overburdened with all that has happened, and it is important to get through it all and grasp the concept of a worthwhile life as quickly and wholeheartedly as they can. As their provider, I am there to support them through this. I am there to answer their questions and to guide them to the many types of assistance that they may need during their cancer journey. Ultimately, the patient will have to come to terms with the concept of living the remainder of their life in a worthwhile fashion. Fortunately, I have found that the majority of my patients are capable of doing this.

As I look back on my experiences caring for patients with a newly diagnosed cancer, I am grateful that I have been able to have been an integral part of their experiences. I am happy that I have been able to successfully guide patients through this very difficult chapter in their lives. I am satisfied that I have done this in a professional manner that makes it easier and more positive for each of them. The patients in my practice, and the experiences that they have had, inspired me many years ago to get involved with local charities, such as Tampa's Faces of Courage and others that exist to lend many types of support to those going through the cancer journey and to those who have survived. I have many meaningful memories of working with all of these affected individuals. It is an honor to have been a part of each patient's experience on their journey. I am indebted to each of them for having allowed me to play the role that I have played.

Reflections On Being A Urologist

By
Kevin O'Kelly, M.D.

Reflections Introduction

My career as a urologist began when I was a young man growing up in Canada. My father had immigrated from Ireland and became a urologist after training at the University of Toronto. My mom was a pediatric nurse who met my father while attending University College Galway. They immigrated from Ireland to Canada and started their new life in 1957. Growing up in a medical environment allowed me to see the joy in practicing medicine. In elementary school and high school, I struggled to be an A student due to my prioritizing sports ahead of academics. My family moved from Toronto to Columbia, SC where I completed high school. I attended the University of South Carolina where I played soccer and obtained a Bachelor of Science Degree in Biology. I attended medical school at St George's University, School of Medicine and completed general surgical residency in Brooklyn, NY followed by a residency in urology at the University of South Florida (USF). At USF, I met Dr. Lester Persky who provided me with the opportunity to become a urologist. Dr. Persky was Professor Emeritus of Urology at Case Western University in Cleveland, OH. and Professor of Urology at USF. He, along with Dr. Jorge Lockhart, trained me to become a urologist. Upon completion of my urology residency I moved to Florence, SC and practiced urology for approximately 30 years.

Being a Urologist.

In May of 1993 I moved from Tampa, FL to Florence, SC and joined a urological practice where I practiced both adult and pediatric urology and treated many types of malignancies. Cancer is a devastating diagnosis that affects not just the patient but also their family, close friends and the medical professionals treating the cancer. Most cancer cases I treated involved prostate cancer.

The diagnosis of prostate cancer begins with a blood test called prostate specific antigen (PSA) which indicates the level of a serine protease in the blood that is elaborated by the epithelial cells of the prostate. The PSA test is nonspecific, but it can be an indicator of possible malignancy. The differential diagnosis of an elevated PSA can include infection, inflammation, enlargement of the prostate, prostate cancer, or prostatic infarction. A urologist becomes involved when the patient is referred by their primary care physician for an elevated PSA. The PSA was never intended to specifically diagnose the presence or absence of prostate cancer but was initially developed to monitor the absence or presence of malignancy after undergoing removal of the prostate gland. The key to success in treating prostate cancer is early diagnosis and treatment.

Prostate Cancer: Diagnosis
When a patient has an elevated PSA, a digital rectal exam (DRE) is performed to evaluate the presence of firmness or irregularity in the prostate. If this is noted, then an MRI of the prostate will be done to delineate the exact size and characteristics of the gland. The radiologists will evaluate for the absence or presence of abnormalities and assign a score of 1 to 5. The higher the score, the greater the risks for clinically significant malignancy. The evaluation is further conducted if the PSA is greater than 10. In that case, the patient will undergo a CT of the abdomen and pelvis and a bone scan. This is called "clinical staging" of the malignancy and will assist in determining the most appropriate forms of treatment for prostate cancer.

There is no absolute uniform treatment for prostate cancer. The treatment needs to be individualized regarding the patient and their desires. When treating newly diagnosed patients. I always try to include the patient, their spouse, and other family members. A cancer diagnosis can be overwhelming, and a family approach is most appropriate to assist the patient along their cancer journey, not only in the diagnosis, but also prognosis, treatment and for supportive care in the future.

Prostate Cancer: Treatment
There are multiple medical and surgical approaches for the treatment of prostate cancer. Surgery is not always indicated, and medical management can assist with the treatment of this disease, which is largely based on staging of the disease. Stages one and two, which are organ confined prostate cancer, are usually treated with surgical intervention. Surgical intervention options include open radical prostatectomy, perineal prostatectomy, laparoscopic

assisted prostatectomy, and robotic prostatectomy. Surgery is not for all patients, in particular patients with stage three and stage 4 adenocarcinoma of the prostate. Stage three disease usually indicates cancer locally outside of the prostate and is best treated with radiation therapy. Radiation therapy now includes External Beam Radiation (EBR) therapy and/or placement of Palladium seeds. Prior to radiation and placement of palladium seeds, a space oar can be placed in the perirectal space to protect the rectum from radiation. Palladium seeds are usually placed by the radiation oncologist with the urologist in the operating room. EBR, which conforms to the size of the gland and surrounding tissue, is performed on an outpatient basis. The dosage of the radiation therapy and frequency of the treatments is determined by the radiation oncologist after consultation with the treating urologist. Patients diagnosed with stage four or metastatic prostate cancer are usually treated with hormonal manipulation which is lowering the amount of circulating testosterone. Testosterone is described as "the fuel to the fire of cancer." Oral agents are available as well as injection therapy for prostate cancer. A medical oncologist may be involved in this portion of the patient's treatment for prostate cancer.

Prostate Cancer: Patient Support
The treatments mentioned above are based solely on urological care for the patient. The human aspect regarding the treatment of prostate cancer is subjective, not objective. With my patients I try to personalize the treatment of prostate cancer. After the initial consultation, I repeat the initial PSA and then have the patient return to the office where I review the repeat PSA in detail including the differential diagnosis. I then prepare the patient for a prostate biopsy. A prostate biopsy can be performed via a transrectal ultrasound of the prostate with guidance or a fusion biopsy of the prostate, where we combine ultrasound and MRI of the prostate with a targeting program. This increases the yield by approximately 10 to 14%.

The most difficult part of treating prostate cancer is when I inform the patient and his family of the diagnosis. As a urologist, I try to be objective but subjective feelings become involved. When taking care of a newly diagnosed cancer patient, some urologists believe and feel that when they tell a patient that they have cancer that they also feel the pain and anguish but will try to remain objective in the presentation of treatments and prognosis as much as possible. As a medical practitioner, I feel sadness in dealing with patients that have high stage disease when the prognosis is not good. I try to be a pillar of strength; however, I also must be honest and realistic. I tell my patients that when they fall, I will pick them up and when they need somebody to lean against, I will be there for them. Patients are usually overwhelmed with the initial diagnosis and have difficulty understanding not only do they have cancer but what is being said after they hear the word "cancer." This is where compassion and empathy become involved. Usually, the spouse is present and is very attentive. I try to read both the patient's facial expressions and tone of voice. This is the place for time and respect. Although we are under pressure to limit time with patients regarding appointments, I always spend that extra time. I encourage the patient and wife to become educated regarding prostate cancer by reviewing the literature about prostate cancer. There are multiple sources of information including journals, textbooks and sometimes the internet. The internet can be a valuable source of finding the correct information (i.e., Mayo Clinic, Johns Hopkins University, Medical University of South Carolina, University of South Florida, Moffitt Cancer Center). I also encourage patients to write down questions on a legal pad to ask me on the next visit. When the patient returns, we discuss the findings of the CT/Bone Scan and then stage the patient. It is at that time we discuss treatment options based on the stage of disease. I always discuss all options of treatment, both surgical and medical, in an unbiased manner.

Helping Patients: Hope and Faith

I always believe that there is hope. Hope in dealing with cancer is an integral part of treatment and having faith that the outcome will be positive, and the cancer will be eradicated. Hope is involved with the daily treatment of cancer at each step of the journey in fighting this dreaded illness. It gives patients the strength to carry on despite treatment issues that will occur at times. Faith is also involved in the treatment of prostate cancer as God has a plan for all. Faith allows the patient faith to deal with reality as well as the future. Informing the patient that their cancer is terminal is based on transparency and honesty. Developing a meaningful life during the diagnosis and treatment. of cancer is especially important. Some medical professionals say quality of life is compromised with the treatment of prostate cancer and any other cancer which is true. How one approaches and deals with these challenges is what makes the journey difficult. Hope is a balance between the present and the future. Hope can change over time with disease progression and management. Hope is an optimistic point of view that can also lead to realism.

This is where I believe support from fellow cancer patients and other support groups make a difference for the recently diagnosed cancer patient. Cancer patients are often unable to discuss their inner feelings, thoughts, and emotions with their physician. Discussing these issues with other patients who have prostate cancer as well as trained professionals can significantly alleviate stress and worry regarding cancer. Prostate cancer in general is a slow growing malignancy although cancer diagnosed in the younger population of men tends to be more aggressive. Prostate cancer is the second most common malignancy in males and in this year alone, there will be approximately 230,000 new diagnoses of prostate cancer and 30,000 deaths in the United States. As with most cancers, early intervention will yield better outcomes in general. Fortunately, there is significant research being conducted to treat prostate cancer providing increased chances of defeating the disease, not only in the United States, but world-wide.

Helping Patients: Saying Goodbye
Saying goodbye is one of the most difficult tasks for a patient who has cancer and for the treating medical professional. A patient's inner circle usually includes spouses, life partners, children, grandchildren, parents, siblings, and close friends.

It is these individuals that we rely on to provide support during this exceedingly difficult journey. If the patient is fortunate to survive this disease, support is essential. As a medical provider, I will discuss the five and seven-year survival rates of malignancy with the patient and members of his support circle, based on staging. These statistical data are based on past and not current or future trends. Each patient is an individual and each has different strengths and weaknesses to fight their cancer.

Helping Patients: Living a Meaningful Life
On a personal note, my father was also a urologist and an excellent surgeon and physician. He was an excellent father who demanded the best out of all three sons. My father was my hero. My father was diagnosed with prostate cancer and lung cancer in 2008. At age 78 his diagnosis was made when he was being treated for diverticulitis with a small rupture. He underwent laparoscopic surgery and during his evaluation was found to have an elevated PSA. The diagnosis of prostate cancer was made, and he elected hormonal manipulation with Casodex over surgery or radiation therapy. He subsequently developed pneumonia and was found to have a left supraclavicular mass which proved to be lung cancer. His nutritional status

was depleted fighting the cancer and he eventually succumbed to the diseases.

My Final Thoughts

As you can see from the above, treatment needs to be tailored to the individual to provide quality of life and satisfaction as determined by each patient's course of therapy. As a urologist we must put aside our scientific mind for our compassionate and empathetic care of the patient.

For those male family members there is a sporadic inheritance of prostate cancer. It would behoove all male family members over age 40 to have a regular PSA test and DRE performed by their primary care physician or urologist. With an early diagnosis we can hopefully alleviate the mortality and morbidity of this disease.

Reflections From An Oncologist

By
Helen Ryan, M.D.

My journey to becoming an oncologist is unique and informs how I think about providing care to a cancer patient. As a young girl I had always wanted to be a doctor. I loved the smell of my pediatrician's office and loved visiting there. My pediatrician was very charming, and I decided that I wanted to be a doctor. I considered doing a pre-med concentration as an undergraduate, but I loved studying literature, so I became an English major instead. After graduating from college, I took a position as a secretary to a Pediatric Hematologist in Boston. Working in that office again sparked my interest in medicine. I began taking classes at a post-baccalaureate program. To gain more experience in the clinical realm I took a position as "Unrelated Bone Marrow Transplant Coordinator." I worked with a team of Bone Marrow Transplant physicians helping to find donors for patients who did not have family donors. It took me four years to complete my studies and I was then accepted to medical school. At that point I was considered an "older" student at 27. My goal was already formed: to become an oncologist with a focus in malignant hematology. And that is what happened. After my training I joined an academic program for two years then moved to Maine and became a malignant hematologist within a private practice.

My focus is on malignant hematology patients which includes a wide variety of diagnoses including lymphoma, leukemia, myeloma. I also see benign hematology patients. I do not treat patients with solid tumor malignancies like breast, lung or colon cancer. My specialty has a wide range of clinical outcomes. Acute leukemia patients are incredibly ill upon presentation and need treatment almost from the moment they are first seen. Unfortunately, a few of them may die prior to the diagnostic work-up being completed. These patients are often seen either directly from the Emergency Department because of how sick they are or are seen in my office because their primary care physician (PCP) calls me directly so they may be seen within 24 hours. My approach to these patients is very different than for those patients who are seen for work-up of abnormal lab findings.

My approach to the acute leukemia patient focuses on stabilization. These patients are often directed to the ER by their PCP's for "abnormal blood counts." Although it may be obvious that they have leukemia, seldom do they hear this from their PCP. Often, I will be the first person to tell them they have leukemia and that this is a life-threatening situation. It is a daunting responsibility and giving that news can be difficult. But having treated many leukemia patients in my career I am able to say with confidence that we will stabilize them and then will have further conversations about their prognosis once we have more data. I can confidently reassure the patients because I know we will have time for more conversations. This experience is difficult for a young doctor fresh out of training but there is a transition that happens as their confidence builds with experience and then becomes reassuring for the patient.

Patients that I see in the outpatient setting span the gamut between those who are quite ill and those with benign issues. The expectations these patients have initially is driven by their PCP's. Some patients have PCP's who are transparent and knowledgeable and tell their patients that they are being seen by me for a suspicion of cancer or for reassurance about a likely benign process. Other patients are unsure why they are being referred to an Oncologist. These patients are understandably extremely nervous being at an Oncology office. That first meeting with the patient may set the tone for the relationship going forward. It is important to "read the room" and to try to gauge where on the spectrum the patient and most likely the family accompanying them are. Doctors want to be reassuring, but if I am concerned that the patient's condition is truly cancer then I am up front during that initial meeting.

Every doctor has a different style. The style of delivery of news and ultimately patient caretaking has developed over the years. My style is straightforward. It is not a style that is universally embraced by other medical providers. Some patients appreciate this. Some patients come to appreciate this style in due course. Other patients are put off completely by this style. I believe this comes in part from the doctor's own personality so is hardwired. Refinement takes place over years of taking care of patients. Doctors initially may try to emulate a mentor's style but eventually the style is burnished until it becomes the doctor's own reflection of her/his personality.

Taking care of many different types of cancer requires shifting gears throughout the clinic day as many different patients are seen. I will see new patients without a diagnosis, new patients with a diagnosis, patients under active treatment, patients who have successfully completed treatment, patients who will remain on treatment for the rest of their lives and patients for whom treatment has not been successful. Each requires a different approach and a different mindset when entering the exam room.

New patients require much time and reassurance from the medical provider. The appointment time is normally an hour. Family members are encouraged to attend as most patients are only able to grasp about fifty percent of what we discuss. My style has been to keep things straightforward. I do not like to discuss "percentages." This can be a difficult concept, but I believe percentages do not apply to single patients.

Patients who do not have a diagnosis pose a unique challenge. I do not want to be overly optimistic as I do not have all or any information about the disease the patient has. I am honest and tell them what steps we will be taking to get to a diagnosis. These patients are the most difficult to see. It is a difficult situation because the diagnosis will take time to complete. Sometimes this can take up to a month and that is a frustrating and nerve-wracking situation for the patient and their loved ones.

Another issue that often comes up in the initial meetings is "Why did I get cancer?" There are very few direct links as to the cause of a patient's cancer outside of tobacco use. I try to explain that I am a physician who treats cancer not a researcher into the causes of cancer. In malignant hematology especially many questions remain unanswered on this front. While I appreciate that this can be a source of frustration and anxiety, I try to concentrate on moving forward to develop the appropriate treatment plan for the patient.

New patients will often seek a second opinion and I encourage all patients to get one. Getting a second opinion is never an insult to the primary oncologist. For someone who works in the medical community, I appreciate the second opinion. It gives me reassurance that I am choosing the correct treatment for my patients. If I have not chosen the correct treatment, then it is a learning experience for me. A second opinion also gives me a resource going forward. If I have a question about another patient, I can reach back out to this expert. Medicine is both an art and a science and there is not always one correct answer. In most cases, we don't know which treatment will provide the best outcome for each individual patient. This is also a lesson in diplomacy and humility. I also value having a second set of eyes on difficult patients. In the community we do not have all the resources that a large academic cancer center can provide for the patient. In my community we do not have access to bone marrow transplantation or car T cell therapy. These therapies can be integral to the treatment of certain cancer types, and I have established a community of referral physicians that I rely upon.

Patients who are starting on a new treatment also require time and reassurance. Patients who are receiving treatment and are being seen for assessment of toxicities are the patients I enjoy seeing the most during my busy days. Any difficulties they may be experiencing are usually conditions we can manage and with which we have had prior experience. The treatment process is the period of trust and relationship building between the patient and the treating physician.

A subset of my patients has incurable cancer which may require either watchful waiting or ongoing treatment. Patients under watchful waiting do not need treatment in the asymptomatic period of their disease because there is no cure. Having the patient go through treatment is not beneficial if they are asymptomatic. The benefit occurs to relieve symptoms. Some of these patients may never require treatment. It seems counterintuitive to not treat cancer but there are asymptomatic patients who do not require any treatment because the toxicity of the treatment is not worth it without clear benefit. This scenario is difficult for some patients who may need to have their anxiety managed.

Patients with incurable cancer sometimes require ongoing maintenance treatment. Once I know that a patient has an incurable cancer, I explain this to them. Patients need as much time as possible to reflect upon this information. These patients usually have an initial intense regimen to gain control of their disease followed by a less intense maintenance treatment. Unfortunately, there will often be side effects from the maintenance treatment. Often these patients will not return to their pre-diagnosis physical well-being and will deal with a lifetime of managing side effects.

Some patients will have a recurrence of the cancer despite initially going into remission. This is a very difficult situation to prepare for and address for the doctor as well as the patient. Patients who present with more advanced disease are more likely to have recurrence of the cancer and in such cases I can try to prepare the patient for this possible outcome. However, even patients who have a 90% cure rate can relapse and recur. Therefore, I tend to shy away from statistics. However, breakthrough therapies are constantly being developed. Several years ago, I had patients who would relapse with lymphoma following stem cell transplant. Many of these patients went on to have experimental therapy with car T cells and were cured. Now this procedure is the standard of care.

There will be patients who succumb to their cancers. Sometimes this happens quickly and other times this happens years later. For me, my long term patients who die from their cancers are emotionally the most difficult. I have followed them and their families for years and have developed close relationships. I want to support the family, but I also need closure. I have attended patient's funerals. As the medical provider, this can be incredibly sad yet emotionally fulfilling.

I have recently left private practice after sixteen years. My new position is a hospital based oncologist taking care of inpatients on a Bone Marrow Transplant and Malignant Hematology Unit. I no longer have long term patients. I do, however, have young acutely ill patients. The relationship is very different than the ones I had with my long term patients. Some of these patients die and my role is to discuss prognosis with the families prior to their passing. Patients can die quickly and sometimes unexpectedly. It is much more difficult as the medical provider because there is no time to prepare patients' families for their loved one's death. Often the family will try to "bargain" asking if there's anything else that can be done. It is heartbreaking and emotionally demanding for me as a medical professional to tell a patient's family and loved ones there is no beneficial treatments left. I do try to honor these patients' and families' journey by reflecting with my colleagues. I remain awed by their love and courage and do what I can to help them to obtain support for the challenges they will face throughout the cancer journey.

Obtaining Support

I rely on help from various colleagues while treating cancer patients. My team includes a Nurse Navigator who is in contact with the patients via phone or portal. The Nurse Navigator guides the patient through the complexities of the health care system and oversees the planning, scheduling and facilitating of daily clinical activities under the supervision of the treating physician. The Nurse Navigator also plays a key role in outlining and explaining the patient's diagnosis and treatment options in accessible terminology. The Nurse Navigator also helps set up appointments for consultation doctor visits such as Radiation Oncology and medical tests. The Navigator can also help with getting financial and social support for the patient.

I have a Nurse Practitioner on the team who shares in the caretaking especially during the active treatment phase. As an inpatient physician I am also training Fellows and Residents. They are a source of rejuvenation for me. Educating the doctors who will follow is a privilege and a reward. I also reach out to my colleagues in physical therapy and nutrition support. Many patients have physical issues due to their cancer or from their treatment. Physical therapists are vital for helping patients regain some of their losses. For help with pain and symptom management, we have palliative care physicians who manage many aspects of this care during treatment, even curative treatment. The Palliative Care team also helps both inpatient and outpatient with the transition to "symptom directed" care only when treatment will no longer be effective. They help with the physical and emotional transition to caring for the dying patient, for the family and the patient.

Additionally, I usually recommend support groups and community groups to help with other aspects of the patient's journey. The support and community groups can also be important for the caregiver. Support for the patient and the caregiver is critical and is a key component of Hope.

Hope

As I previously noted, I do not like to quote statistics. I do consider it important to give reasons to hope for patients. If it is reasonable to expect recovery or even cure rom the cancer, I discuss this frequently with patients especially when patients are feeling overwhelmed or discouraged. Even patients with incurable cancers have reason to hope. I believe it is important to discuss that patients with incurable cancer have a chronic disease. Patients with other chronic diseases will not have a cure. It is important for patients

to know that some days will be better than others and I want them to
them to understand that there will be days, maybe weeks, or even months
that they will not think about their diagnosis. This hope needs to be tied to
realistic expectations and I try to be mindful of a patient's goals and discuss
if they are realistic. For example, a patient wanting to run a marathon may
be realistic in some cases but in others it will not. In those in whom this is
not realistic a discussion about more realistic goals is needed. Maybe a 10K
is a better goal. Hope is vitally important for the patient, but it cannot be
unrealistic, and there may come a time when it is necessary to accept the
reality and prepare to say good-bye.

Saying Good-bye

Of course, this is the most difficult conversation to have with patients and
their families. I feel strongly that the patient needs to be told when there is
nothing left to offer so they can spend whatever time they have left in the
way that they choose. I discuss with the patient their preferences for where
they would like to be to say their good-byes. There are patients who wish
to fight until the end despite the inevitable. These patients usually die in
the hospital. We try to make that experience as comforting as possible by
putting a patient in a large room where the family can visit and be present for
the end. We as medical providers only intervene with measures that provide
comfort. In young patients sometimes the parents or family will not want
them to be told that the end is near. All patients, though, are aware when
the end is near, often even before the family. If the preference is for a death
at home, we then involve hospice services that provide care in the home.
In addition, hospice will provide supportive services including social work,
spiritual counseling, and bereavement counseling. I do not advise patients
how to say good-bye, but I do try to respect their wishes for the setting in
which they wish to have their good-byes. It is difficult to prepare to say goodbye, but there are opportunities for each patient to spend their remaining
time living a meaningful life.

A Meaningful Life

As a doctor I do not feel I have the authority to tell people how to live a
meaningful life. Every patient is different. Every patient has different spiritual
beliefs. My experience has been that when a patient knows that their life is
going to be abbreviated this puts a magnifying lens on the remaining time.
My role is to try to give the patient an idea what that time course looks like.
Of course, we as doctors do not always know but it is unfair to give false
hope. As I have said, my style is to be extremely open and honest. Patients

especially with incurable but indolent type cancer can do well for a very long-time. Clinically, though, abrupt changes can occur, and a patient may become acutely ill and sometimes die. Those situations are difficult to prepare for. Always being present and listening to the patient and their family is key at every appointment. Making the patient feel valued is vitally important. Listening to the choices the patient is making and being affirming is how I see my role in supporting a meaningful life.

It has been the honor of a lifetime to work with my patients and be part of their journey. I have had the privilege of seeing people at their most vulnerable. This is the most humbling and joyful part of my chosen career. One of the most rewarding parts of my career is helping patients understand their complicated illness and to help them navigate the complex and often confusing world of our health care system. My patients' and families' courage at all stages of their cancer journeys provides me with the inspiration and fortitude to continue the battle against cancer. My success is measured by my ability to make their journeys more tolerable and to respect and honor their wishes no matter what the outcome may be.

Caring for the Mental Health Needs of Patients with Cancer: A Psychosocial Oncologist

By
Timothy Steinhoff, M.D.

Taking care of patients in an honor and a privilege; there is a level of trust and respect afforded to physicians that is not given to others. As a psychiatrist, I learn about my patients' most difficult experiences and challenging dynamics with a fully vested faith that with this knowledge I will care for them with dignity and respect. Finally, as a psycho-oncologist, a psychiatrist who specializes in the care of patients with cancer, I travel with my patients on their journey across the care continuum from diagnosis, through treatment, into survivorship, through the difficulties of relapse, and ultimately reaching end of life. Bearing witness and partaking in the expedition allows me to troubleshoot problems, challenge maladaptive ways of thinking, and attempt to reframe what lies ahead.

The mental healthcare for a patient with cancer is no more or less important than it is for any patient. Simply put, it is essential. A cancer diagnosis is a life-changing event that brings challenges that are similar in some ways and significantly different in others when contrasted with other medical illnesses. Unlike a new diagnosis of diabetes, high cholesterol, or hypertension, cancer brings a weight felt like few other conditions. The gravity is experienced through the historical lens of a cancer diagnosis in which a death sentence was assured. For a great part of medical history, the diagnosis was not even shared with patients for fear that they would lose hope and ability to cope. Families would contribute to the secrecy, minimizing the experience of the patient, and withholding information from other loved ones; for the diagnosis was stigmatized and shameful. In some cultures, information is still withheld to this day.

We as a medical community contributed to this. We recommended silence. We modeled behaviors of dismissal. Even as support groups emerged for colon cancers, head and neck cancers, and breast cancer, patients were discouraged by their doctors from participating. The idea of these groups was met with hostility by the medical community; the benefits were not seen. In fact, it has only been about 60 years since the taboo of talking about death with cancer patients was challenged by psychiatrist Elizabeth Kubler-Ross. This history and how we as a medical community have interacted with the disease and the patients and families affected by it, casts a long shadow. The emergence of psychosocial oncology as a specialty of psychiatry began in the 1970s and has blossomed into a robust and vibrant field today that continues to grow, learn, and adapt. It is with an understanding of the history and the training and work as a psycho-oncologist, that I engage patients.

I meet patients in the cancer center in the same clinic they see their medical oncologists, radiation oncologists, surgeons, palliative care physicians, and nurses. It is where they get their blood drawn and where they sit for infusions. Patients check in at the same desk and often have their vitals taken by the same medical assistants when they come to see a psychiatrist as they do when they have an appointment for a chemotherapy infusion. This is all done purposefully. I believe this reflects both the importance of mental health care and the progress that has been made with regards to the stigma psychiatric treatment carries.

Much is the same during an initial appointment with a patient who has cancer as would be done in a general outpatient psychiatry clinic. I inquire about current symptoms, historical symptoms, previous treatment, medical and psychiatric history, family and social histories, and conduct a mental status exam. There are some unique and cancer-specific questions I ask and areas I query:

Can you tell me about your cancer?
What symptoms did you notice before you were diagnosed with cancer?
Where were you when you were told about your diagnosis?
Who were you with when you found out?
How did you feel when you heard the diagnosis?

I start open-ended and allow the conversation to go where the patient takes it. As they tell me about their experience, I am listening for the answers to the follow up questions. When the information does not arise spontaneously, I ask.

I look to understand what symptoms presented before and leading up to the diagnosis so that if the patient experiences them again, we can connect physical symptoms to psychological experiences; new anxiety or panic for example. A patient with colon cancer who noticed pain and constipation with bowel movements before diagnosis and now experiencing constipation during treatment because of opioid medications might have unexplained anxiety symptoms driven by an unconscious connection of the physical symptom and worries that the cancer has returned. Being aware can help to raise these to consciousness.

Knowing where patients were, who they were with, and what they felt when they learned of their disease can be incredibly revealing and offers a wealth of knowledge. While it feels like I have heard it all, I know I will continue to be amazed by the variety of answers. While I am not the oncologist, and not the physician that shares the diagnosis with patients, I still feel sadness for what immediate access to medical record information has resulted in. There was once a time when the oncologist would receive the radiology report and pathology results enabling them to incorporate this information clinically and present it to the patient in a thoughtful manner. Patients now have access to test results, pathology reports, and chart notes instantly; often reading the diagnostic information before the oncologist has had a chance to, in the midst of busy clinic days. Many patients have told me how difficult it was to see the information and feel lost, waiting for the chance to talk to their oncologist about what the results mean and what the next steps are.

Can you tell me about your treatment so far?
What are the next steps in your treatment?
These questions aim to address a few things. I want to understand how the patient appreciates their diagnosis and treatment as well as what they expect of it. It allows for major discrepancies between what the oncologist is discussing (e.g., palliative chemotherapy) vs the patient's expression of what that means (e.g., curative chemotherapy). It alerts me to ask more questions and encourage them to talk further with their oncologist. Getting a sense of how treatment is going also clues me in to symptoms that I might be able to target with my toolbox of psychotropic medications. These can include

pre-treatment anxiety, claustrophobia during scans or radiation treatments, nausea, poor sleep, and the list goes on.

Who are you responsible for?
Who do you lean on for support?
Knowing this helps to establish what a patient's support circle looks like. These will be the people that bring them to appointments, sit with them at infusion, bring meals, watch movies, laugh, cry, and gossip. When there is a limited support group, I might encourage ways that patients can expand their social circle whether through support groups, re-engaging in hobbies they have dropped. Equally as important is identifying who patients care for. Not only because it can impact the decisions they make about their treatment but are important in legacy which I will discuss in the chapter on meaning.

Who were you before your diagnosis, who are you now, and who do you want to be?
A cancer diagnosis can make patients forget the life they have lived, the life they want to live, and the way they are living now. I like to delineate this timeline for them to hand control back to them. While a cancer diagnosis is life-changing, that change is up to the patient.

What are you most fearful of?
What are you most hopeful for?
The themes of fears and hopes are centered around the cancer diagnosis the great majority of the time. Most might expect that the answers would be: fearful of dying and hopeful for cure. However, just as each person is an individual, each answer is unique. I listen intently for the fears – these will drive feelings and emotions about treatment and give information about how and where the patient may be suffering (something I will touch on in a later chapter). They also allow a peak into previous experiences with difficult situations. Hopes outline sources of strength and courage. Hope reveals priorities, goals, and dreams. I hold onto these, they are helpful when reframing difficult time-points in treatment and shape how I will work with the patient.

Follow up appointments are multi-fold in nature. They serve as an opportunity to check in with how treatments are progressing and how the patient is adjusting to the diagnosis and interventions. They also act as medication assessments to determine effect, response, side effects, or need for adjustments. Follow up appointments are also a time for me to continue to get to know my patients and work with them in a holistic fashion. I look to incorporate the following themes into our visits:

What are you most proud of so far in life?
A cancer diagnosis can act as a vacuum that draws the air out of a room; a switch that turns the light off. I am eager to learn what ignites the flame inside my patients, what they have accomplished, and what has been important to them. I reach for this later when we talk about legacy building.

What makes a "good" life?
What makes a "good" death?
Mortality is a difficult topic to discuss and unless imminent, not a topic I bring up in the first few appointments unless the patient does. However, as our treatment relationship together grows, I do start to reflect with them on what constitutes a "good" life. These attributes are important in working with patients as they make decisions through their cancer treatment course. When they feel as though things are approaching a fork in the road and they are not sure which path to go down, we can look back on the characteristics of what they believe makes a good life and draw up a list of what the available options offer. These ideas hold true when talking about a "good" death. It may seem odd to talk about having a good death, but it is frankly quite important. While difficult to think about, particularly in the context of why patients are seeing me, it is fair to argue that everybody dies, so everybody can think about what it means to have a good death. This is often how I present it to patients. When not faced with imminent death, patients can often provide thoughtful engagement on this. When it is too difficult to talk about it with regards to themselves, I encourage them to talk about what these concepts would mean for those they love.

What has changed in life for the better since your diagnosis?
Since your diagnosis, what has changed that you would change again?
These questions are designed to reframe what is typically discussed with a negative valence with a positive edge. While it can be rather surprising for patients to be asked to think about what has improved in their life, it does help challenge black and white thinking to appreciate some of the shades of gray. Perhaps relationships have grown in a positive way, or being out of work has allowed them to spend more time on a hobby. I incorporate a conversation about what has changed that they wish could go back to as it was or, perhaps, change in a way that is new and different. This is really a way of asking, "what has changed that you do not like" while framing it as an

opportunity for further change and improvement. The answers I have heard to this have included nuanced topics from relationships to practical frustrations like the way a favorite food tastes.

What legacy do you want to live now?
What legacy do you want to leave?
The impact that one leaves through the way they live their life today, and the impression on others that will carry on after death can be difficult topics to discuss, but integral to a patient's dignity. I will discuss legacy further in the chapter on Living a Meaningful Life.

Obtaining Support
Buttressing: Sources of Support
The vast majority of the time, when patients are meeting me, there has been an identified need for additional support. Sometimes it is a patient that seeks out the care, sometimes it is at the behest of family or friends, and other times the patient's primary treatment team. I talk with patients about the importance of finding support and a few core sources: self, friends and family, community, treatment team, and support groups.

Self
Learning how to rely on one's self, particularly during a difficult time such as a cancer diagnosis and treatment, is akin to building a foundation. While, those around us are important and vital supports, in order to benefit fully, we must be able to depend on ourselves. Some of the ways I encourage patients to build self-esteem and self-reliance involve mindfulness meditations, yoga, art therapies, spiritual practices, medications, and individual therapy.

I use the category of mindfulness meditations to include exercises including deep breathing, grounding exercises, progressive muscle relaxation, guided imagery, and mindfulness proper. The benefits of mindfulness are well-described in the medical literature. There are many resources I talk about with patients, many of which are free and easily accessible online or through smartphone or tablet apps. I tell patients the only true cost is their time. When I meet with patients, I encourage commitment to mindfulness activities for as little as five minutes every day. I describe the skills developed are like building muscle; it is necessary to exercise and practice to strengthen and grow. While it may seem tempting to reach for the mindfulness skills only when feeling stressed, anxious, sad, angry, or overwhelmed, it is really quite difficult to effectively use the tools when you have not trained using them when feeling well. I encourage patients to practice mindfulness as one of the first activities of the day. By the end of the day, making an excuse that you will "just do it tomorrow" is all too convenient.

To demonstrate how easy and painless this is, I will often guide a patient through an activity during a session. One of my favorites is titled Leaves on a stream. In this exercise, you are encouraged to close your eyes and envision sitting on a grassy hill under a tree next to a flowing stream. The stream has leaves floating on the surface that move with the water. This scene provides a visual allowing you to place your thoughts on leaves and watch them drift down stream. There are no "good" or "bad" thoughts, just thoughts. You do not dwell on them, simply let them come into your mind, deposit them on a leaf, and watch them move along. The same principle holds true for feelings – acknowledge, deposit, and drift. When I ask patients to tell me what the experience was like and what they noticed, I hear common themes: it was not as hard as they thought it would be, it was relaxing, they felt their breathing and heart rate slow. This is buy-in and I ask them to commit to doing it a few times a week until we see each other again. Firming these skills increases self-reliance.

For some, the thought of sitting calmly, breathing deeply, and visualizing is not appealing. For those who find therapy in moving, I will encourage yoga or Tai chi.

Music therapy and art therapy come in many genres, colors, themes, and shades. For some, this can be coloring or paint-by-number and for others, dabbling with a musical instrument they last picked up in primary school. Some may use composing a musical piece as a means of expressing internal thoughts and feelings and others might take to a canvas to represent anxiety, fears, or hopes. I find having patients bring their pieces into session to share, an incredibly rich topic for conversation. I have had patients who make candles with scents that remind them of places they have been, scents that have helped to alleviate nausea or relax them in the evening. I recently had a patient who made candles with scents she felt represented different members of her care team and another who brought in jewelry she has made with themes representing different stages of her treatment. These activities are relaxing, distracting, engaging, and build self-esteem.

For those who find importance in spiritual and religious practices, I will encourage them to remain engaged. In the cancer center at my institution, we have spiritual care practitioners who meet with patients. The patients who find spirituality to be integral to their life, will often find meaning, esteem, and strength.

As a psychiatrist, one of the tools in my toolbox is medication, and I think of medications just in this way: as an instrument. I am clear with patients that medications are not a "fix" and have limitations. They are intended to enhance the efforts and work the patient is doing. This being said, there is absolutely a time, place, and need for medication. Whether it be disabling anxiety preventing someone from being able to tolerate imaging scans, radiation treatments, or chemotherapy infusions, or depression that makes getting out of bed impossible, taking care of basic needs, with feelings of hopelessness and worthlessness, debilitating. Medications can be essential in helping patients realize and actualize their potential.

Finally, and perhaps most important (this may be biased), is encouraging patients to engage in individual therapy. While we have come quite a distance in destigmatizing mental health care, and many famous people talk about their own experiences with therapy, I still find that patients withdraw when I discuss the benefits of individual therapy. While there are too many modalities to dive into here, and doing so would be beyond the scope of this chapter, I will discuss therapy with each patient the first time I meet them. I try to dispel the Hollywood portrayal of the Freudian couch and the distant therapist biting the ear piece of his glasses. Therapy is an opportunity for patients to explore themselves, their thoughts and feelings, and think of ways they can incorporate these insights into working towards being the person they want to be and live the way they hope to live. When I am met with a "no," I tell them, "that is fine. I hear you saying not now." As I continue to meet with them, I will offer the option again.

Friends and family
I spend a great deal of time with patients understanding their support network. This includes friends, family, and community (discussed next). Having just highlighted many ways that patients with cancer can bolster their self-support, being able to rely on others is an important factor in moving through their cancer treatment journey. It can be exceptionally hard for patients to ask for help since the mere need to ask gives truth and reality to their cancer. I will have patients trade roles and tell me how they would

want to help if it was someone they cared about walking in their shoes. It can be effective to break down practical and emotional needs and how to ask for those to be met. Recognizing that some people might be ideal for reliable transportation and meals while others better for coffee, stories, and distraction can be a valuable approach for patients to think about ways to incorporate those around them in their care.

For many, engaging family can mean returning to roles that everyone has already transitioned out of (parent-child, older sibling-younger sibling, etc.) and it can feel like a regression to hold those positions again. In some circumstances, there may be a premature advancement in the situation where a child cares for a parent who would otherwise not yet need late-life care and support. Labeling and acknowledging these feelings can be helpful in understanding why the roles can be difficult to accept, making them a little more tolerable.

I would be remiss not to acknowledge how support roles can shift when one enters remission or survivorship. There is often an abrupt forced normalization in which expectations of and for patients move towards the "old normal." Family returns to previous roles and friends look for the friendship to be as it once was. It is important to talk with patients about this, help set expectations, and discuss ways to talk with those they care about. Continued support may be needed; albeit in different ways.

Community (social clubs, faith/religion, work)
Community outside of close family and friends can be an incredible source of support during and after cancer treatment. For some patients, a cancer diagnosis can induce reflexive withdrawal from spending time with their community. This may be because it feels too difficult to talk about the diagnosis and treatment. It is very reasonable to need space and an adjustment period after learning of a difficult, life-changing diagnosis before sharing with others. However, for some patients this becomes the default mode of interacting with those around them. As discussed previously, talking about it can make the illness real. Patients fear those around them will view them different a child cares for a parent who would otherwise not yet need late-life care and support. Labeling and acknowledging these feelings can be helpful in understanding why the roles can be difficult to accept, making them a little more tolerable.

I would be remiss not to acknowledge how support roles can shift when one enters remission or survivorship. There is often an abrupt forced normalization in which expectations of and for patients move towards the "old normal." Family returns to previous roles and friends look for the friendship to be as it once was. It is important to talk with patients about this, help set expectations, and discuss ways to talk with those they care about. Continued support may be needed; albeit in different ways.

Community (social clubs, faith/religion, work)
Community outside of close family and friends can be an incredible source of support during and after cancer treatment. For some patients, a cancer diagnosis can induce reflexive withdrawal from spending time with their community. This may be because it feels too difficult to talk about the diagnosis and treatment. It is very reasonable to need space and an adjustment period after learning of a difficult, life-changing diagnosis before sharing with others. However, for some patients this becomes the default mode of interacting with those around them. As discussed previously, talking about it can make the illness real. Patients fear those around them will view them differently – see them as too 'sick' to participate in work events, not 'strong enough' to handle projects. It becomes easier to attempt to hide the information so as not to have to explain over and over. However, most patients find that their colleagues are a source of support and encouragement. Yes, there will be times that side effects of treatment, or the disease itself will necessitate time away from work, but when co-workers understand the reason, they are often eager to accommodate. Additionally, having a group of people that one spends their professional life with offers a different quality of support than what family and close friends provide; and often a distraction from routine day-to-day life.

For those who are active in a faith or religion, there can be difficult questions that arise in the context of the disease diagnosis. A life-threatening illness may challenge a patient's faith and raise existential questions. I encourage patients to look for answers instead of closing doors. This can be done through spiritual care services in our cancer center, or by seeking out members of their community.

Treatment team

As cancer treatment options and therapeutic complexity have increased, so too has the composition of the treatment team taking care of them. What was once only an oncologist, now commonly includes a medical oncologist, surgical oncologist, radiation oncologist, supportive and palliative care, psychosocial oncology/psycho-oncology, social work, spiritual care, and a myriad of complementary and alternative therapies. Each member of the team has strengths they bring to the table in supporting the patient as a whole person. Cancer centers are much better resourced than they once were and this allows us to support patients in many different ways. I analogize cancer treatment to a triathlon where different legs of the race require different skills and training. Each member of the treatment team is a specialist in a different aspect of the race; we work as a team to navigate the course towards a shared goal of reaching the finish line.

Support groups

Cancer and survivorship support groups provide a venue for patients to hear from others that are walking or have walked the same path. It is one thing to hear words of support from friends, family, co-workers, the treatment team, but these same words can transcend into solidarity when hearing them from someone with the same scars and wounds. There is an amazing sense of camaraderie in support groups. There are many different types of support groups that range from general to cancer-specific. Some support groups focus on particular issues encountered in cancer such as anxiety or grief. Many national cancer organizations facilitate support groups and networks that allow patients to interact with a diverse group of people from across the country. I make a point to educate patients about the purpose and format of these groups because I find that many patients hear support group and envision group therapy. While I can share many positives about standard group therapy, it is an entirely different format. There is a long history of support groups for patients undergoing cancer treatment, and the longevity speaks to the important role they serve.

I have covered some of the fundamental ways that I encourage patients to find support. The architects of many historical buildings dating to the age of antiquity, and earlier, understood the need for buttressing; a structure cannot stand without support. Just as these complex architectural feats needed support, so do our patients.

Hope

Hope: Active, Affective, Achievable

Hope is incredibly nuanced and difficult to define succinctly. We understand the hope for a tasty dessert is different from hoping the weather is sunny is different from hoping that cancer treatment is successful. Nevertheless, we use the same word. Hope at its core is a cognitive framework, heavily laden with affect and emotion, with a goal that is – actually or theoretically – achievable. A loss of hope, or hopelessness, would then suggest that the idea of achieving the goal has dwindled or disappeared. It might be easy to see then that this can be a feedback loop in which seeing progress towards the goal can increase the hope to achieve it, and a lack of progress, or feeling as though the goal line is moving out of reach, can deplete the hope of getting there.

Hope is distinct from positivity and optimism. Colloquially, we might use these terms interchangeably, but I think it is important to understand the subtleties of each. I make the distinction because patients can experience negative feelings about their diagnosis and treatment and still hold hope: they need to know this. It can be incredibly difficult to "stay positive" following a cancer diagnosis; there is an immense amount of unnecessary stress patients put on themselves to remain in this mindset. It can be frustrating for patients to hear "be optimistic," from friends, family, colleagues, and their treatment team. It suggests that existing in any other way, is wrong. Additionally, forcing an optimistic framework necessitates positive outcomes. This is a setup for disappointment, discouragement, and despair. Rather, I encourage patients to live with a sense of hope. To let hope guide their path.

Hope is a desire for something to happen. It is a focus on the future, a forward mindset. It shifts through treatment. Hopes at the time of diagnosis are different than hopes as treatment begins, and as one enters survivorship. Each step along the way necessitates a resetting and recalibrating. Hope is an active process; it cannot be done passively and hope does not happen to us or for us.

Hope has been implicated in better psychological resilience in patients coping with cancer. Patients with high hope measures, have been reported to experience pain to a lesser degree, report better physical health, and express higher levels of positive emotions than patients with low hope measures.

What are you hopeful for?

When I sit with patients, I will ask them what they are hopeful for. This allows me the opportunity to hear both what is important to them as well as how they view their cancer diagnosis. Certainly, a statement such as "I am hopeful to see my daughter get married this fall," is much different than "I am hopeful to see my newborn grandchild graduate from college." Starting the conversation helps me gauge the way the patient understands the impact their cancer diagnosis will have on them. It also opens the conversation to think about other hopes such as hoping to enjoy quality time with loved ones watching a movie and sharing dinner.

Hope does not reject truth. This is important. When having difficult conversations with patients about the state of their health and the realities they face, we need to offer hope while accepting and acknowledging the facts. Helpful ways to incorporate this in a clinical context can be to say, "I am hoping with you and…" where what follows is often "we need to prepare for," or "we need to understand," or "the current state is." I am deliberate in reminding patients that I hope alongside them. I do. This again illustrates that hope is active, goal-directed, and rich with emotion and affect.

I mentioned in the previous chapter, that I ask patients what they are most hopeful for. It can be helpful for patients to break down large, nebulous hopes into tangible goals that can be achieved. I also find it beneficial to ask patients what they can be hopeful about even if they feel that being hopeful about their cancer is fruitless. Identifying hopes with more imminent goals and time points can facilitate the positive feedback I discussed previously. Hoping to enjoy going to the beach with friends and family this upcoming weekend and hoping to relish the time with grandchildren after school this week are opportunities to see hopes become reality. Slowing down and identifying these can be helpful for patients to realize there is much to be hopeful for.

Saying Goodbye

Saying Goodbye: Reflecting on a Life Lived

What does it mean to say goodbye? There are countless ways and situations in which we bid farewell to others. At times, we intend for it to punctuate a brief period, and at others there is a permanence. Different cultures and languages have phrases intended to deliver the meaning of each. Some cultures, the Hawaiian language for instance, use the same words for hello and goodbye. As children, we learn to wish a good day to our parents when we go off to school, say goodbye to friends at the end of the school day, and goodnight before bed. As we get older, friends move away, perhaps we go off to college, and with each of these milestones in life, we mark endings and new beginnings. That is what goodbye is after all, the punctuation at the end of a chapter before turning the page to start the next.

For patients with cancer, there are many goodbyes. Some are joyous and others are sad. There are the endings of surgeries, infusions, and interventional treatments. The conclusions of these chapters, are often exciting and marked with celebration. At my institution, the radiation oncology department holds a graduation ceremony when a patient completes their grueling course of treatment. This goodbye is marked with pomp and circumstance.

Other endings can be more difficult. Patients often develop a close relationship with the nurses that work in the infusion center, who see them at each session, and are by their side for the long hours of treatments. When treatment ends, the abrupt cessation of those touchpoints can be jarring; the goodbye hard. Another difficult goodbye can be to another patient who sat in an infusion chair nearby, in the waiting room, or participated in a shared support group. These goodbyes can be for many reasons. Sometimes it is because the other patient has completed treatment and entered remission. However, loss can also be a reason and sometimes the person who sat in the pod next door passed away.

The death of another patient is difficult. It is again a reminder of the real nature of the diagnosis and possible outcomes. Patients I work with who describe the difficulty with the loss of another patient they became close to will often jump to the conclusion they will have the same happen to them. I remind them that each person's treatment course is unique.

Thinking about goodbyes is a time for reflection. The retrospection is not only for the time between diagnosis and today, but for their entire life. This means thinking about who they want to be able to say goodbye to and how to say it. While these conversations can be incredibly hard, I have found that when patients have the opportunity to consider who they would like to have time to talk to and say goodbye to, they feel a sense of closure that otherwise would have been missing. Pausing to think about who these people are, and mentally (or physically) writing a list can be helpful. It is important to note, and I reflect this with patients, that closure does not necessarily mean speaking to or meeting with the person they want to say farewell to. For some, fractured relationships, strained dynamics, and great time and distance since last meaningful encounters can make direct contact difficult – both for the patient and the other party involved. Closure can also come through other methods such as writing a letter, journaling, or discussing in therapy.

Preparing for goodbye is a time to finish unfinished work. In psychological terms, unfinished business is about working on tasks that have been avoided because of interpersonal and emotional impacts that are feared. In some circles, unfinished work brings existential guilt. Resolving the unfinished business can lead to a sense of peace. From a grief and bereavement standpoint, it is thought that dealing with unfinished work is integral to the process of mourning the loss. These themes come in many flavors and varieties, unique to each patient. Often, these naturally emerge during conversations about death and dying. If specific tasks do not bubble to the surface, the feelings and emotions often do. I provide space for the patient to explore those and contemplate them and bear witness to the experience.

In practical terms, unfinished business extends beyond the standard psychological meaning to include pragmatic and theoretical future matters that are still unresolved. For some, these goals are milestones in the lives of people they love such as weddings, graduations, anniversaries, and reunions. For others, it is completing an endeavor such as a writing piece, a carpentry project, or volunteer activity. Patients may describe a loss of motivation to complete these tasks. Talking about why the project is meaningful to them can serve as an inspiration to continue the work. Identifying this unfinished business and planning ways to work on it can alleviate angst that patients may not even be aware is tied to the activity.

Thus far, I have focused on saying goodbye to others, and would be remiss not to discuss the difficult task of saying goodbye to one's self. I do not mean this in the literal sense of course, but rather the symbolic act of grieving the loss of life one has lived and the future opportunities that one will be unable to see. While the theory of stages of grief have oscillated in and out of vogue over the years, I think it is helpful to conceptualize the work patients do in the process of grieving their loss. Often the first state experienced is that of denial – many times initiated by a strong sense of shock at the time of diagnosis. Here, inability to accept the fate of death is experienced. Anger is the next stage marked by with frustration and irritability. Here we see questions like "why me" and feelings that it is "not fair." This state may be what first sets off a referral to psychiatry. The emotions can be difficult for the oncology team to sit with and reflect. It is important not to stymie these feelings. Bargaining is described as the next state of grief in which patients will attempt to negotiate, ask for remission of symptoms, for additional time. Often, what is bargained for is linked with some of the hopes and unfinished work we have previously discussed. Sadness and depression come next, and for patients that were not referred in the anger phase and show prominent symptoms of depression, the referral to psychiatry occurs here; affect is described as sullen and despair intrudes. Acceptance is when patients have reached a psychological place of embracing the reality they face and feel a sense of peace.

As patients move through these states of grief it is imperative to understand that they are not unidirectional or linear. For example, denial might present in the clinic room on the day of diagnosis and then again when faced with the difficult conversation that the disease has progressed through multiple lines of therapy and further cancer-directed treatment options are unavailing. The return to denial may be followed by a restoration to a place of acceptance if meaningful work had been previously done.

Developing A Meaningful Life
Search for Meaning: The Journey to a Meaningful Life
Many existential philosophers, psychologists, and psychiatrists have explored the concept of meaning. Finding meaning, or at least thinking about it is not unique to those with a cancer diagnosis. However, a cancer diagnosis, often compels a patient to search and reflect. I utilize the concepts described by psychiatrist and Holocaust survivor Viktor Frankl in his development of logotherapy and the more recently structured group and individual meaning centered therapy in my work.

What is meaning?

We start with a shared, common belief that life has meaning, or at least has the potential for meaning. Universally, we therefore have both a need for meaning and the opportunity to search for and find it. Meaning is derived from a focus outward on goals, achieving tasks, tending to responsibilities, and building relationships rather than an inward focus on suffering, pain, and the illness. The importance in human existence is demonstrated by our search of meaning, connection of meaning, and creation of meaning.

What brings meaning?

"He who has a why to live can bear almost any how." – Friedrich Nietzsche

In searching for meaning, we look to our past and present selves while thinking about who and what we want our future self to be. Our attitudes and outlook on life impact our identification of meaning. For some this can be feeling the pride of making it to weekly chemotherapy treatments, "surviving" a family gathering, or the happiness of watching a child meet a milestone. The life roles we hold and transition through as well as the work we do bring a sense of meaning. These can be the role of child, sibling, parent, cousin, grandparent, friend, co-worker. Meaning derived from each of these roles brings different value through the lifespan. Finally, the experiences we have in life offer a source of meaning. These include relationships we have, spiritual experiences and connections, as well as relatedness to the world and nature around us. Meaning comes from the experience of these relationships. This can be with other people, pets, engaging in painting or music, or witnessing and partaking in the beauty of nature. Our values, attitudes, roles, and experiences, impart purpose and worth in a meaningful life. Pulling from these, hopefully allows for the development of resources – a collection of skills and source of resolve – to draw from for meaning.

Meaning and identity BC and AD

I ask patients to tell me who they were before cancer (BC) and who they think they are today, after diagnosis (AD). It is often quite easy for people to tell me who they were before the diagnosis. When I ask them who they are now, the almost universal answer for patients struggling psychologically is "I do not know." I use the information they gave me about how they viewed who they were before the diagnosis to ask how they might be the same or different now. Surprising most, is the fact that many of these aspects of their identity are the same. They are still a parent/sibling/child, they identify with their role at work, and the hobbies they enjoy. What might have changed is their ability to do the things they used to do that allowed for easy identification with that role or taking part in that experience. This is where I will challenge them to think about how they can continue to be the role they identify with by "doing" it in a different way. Here, the distinction between "doing" and "being" is made. There are many ways to do a task necessary to be the identity we connect with. For example, someone struggling with identifying as being a parent for their child because of fatigue from treatments, may identify the meaningful way they did parenting as coaching the softball team and coordinating the after-game celebration. Thinking about doing parenting by being present at the game and cheering from the stands as an equally important way of being a parent can be a helpful reframe.

Suffering
"To live is to suffer, to survive is to find some meaning in the suffering." – Friedrich Nietzsche

It seems odd to include suffering in a conversation of meaning amongst other topics such as identity and legacy, but suffering is a part of every life. We all experiencing suffering on a spectrum spanning from negligible to overwhelming. The control we have over how we chose to respond to these situations, the attitude we bring to the table, is what permits us to survive. For many patients they will describe the diagnosis and treatment of cancer as the greatest suffering they have experienced in life. For some, far fewer, they will share that they have "been through worse." Regardless of past experiences with suffering, there is opportunity to find meaning in the experience.

Legacy
Legacy lived – We are the summation of our past and present experiences. The past is not limited to solely that which we have individually experienced, but rather the shared human history we have in common both on a world-wide scale and within our families and communities. The patient's personal story includes accomplishments, their family story, what they have learned, and the roles they have held. This is the legacy they are living; this is what has brought meaning to their life.

Legacy left – We leave a legacy behind that becomes part of the legacy lived for those around us. It is incredibly powerful to be in control of the legacy that one leaves behind. In discussing what we refer to as "legacy work," we think about ways that patients can leave a piece of themselves in a meaningful way for those they care about and love. Legacy work has many variations and is unique to each patient. For some, it is composing a letter, for others it is writing a book. I encourage thinking about ways that they can participate in future events that they will not be able to attend such as graduations, weddings, anniversaries. Making a video to be played, leaving a letter to be read, or imparting an object for the event are all ways this can be done. We reflect on the values, attitudes, roles, and experiences and think of ways these can be represented for others. I worked with a carpenter who left his toolbox for his children so they could experience the activities that were so important to his identity. I worked with a musician who composed a piece to be played at her child's wedding. I had the opportunity to sit with grandparents who put together photo albums and cookbooks so that traditions that have been held by them can be carried forward by the next generation.

Our search for meaning is never done, but this does not imply that we never find it. Meaning is not found in pot of gold at the end of a rainbow, but rather discovered and experienced in the journey there.

Providing Care for Cancer Patients

By
Raymond Thomason, III, M.D.

I am honored for the invitation to share my experience of 36 years providing care for my dear patients, friends, and family grappling with that dreaded six-word disease that no one ever wants to hear - CANCER.

I began the practice of medicine in 1976 after completing medical school, followed a residency in Internal Medicine and a fellowship in Gastroenterology and Hepatology. After many years of training, I started a private medical practice as a gastroenterologist and hepatologist - a liver specialist. A large part of my practice involved the diagnosis and treatment of various cancers: esophageal, gastric, colon, pancreas, and liver cancer.

Before I share my approach to cancer, it is important that I provide you the backdrop of my experience with cancer. My story involves not only the journey of my patients but is heavily weighted with the cancer journeys of members of my family, friends, and myself. The cancer journey has taught me much about the humanity of man: the frailty and fear, the strength and courage, the kindness and empathy of strangers, and the beauty and the resilience of the human spirit despite the reality of dealing with one's own mortality. Each patient has taught me something that I have carried forward to the next patient.

My initial exposure to cancer occurred when I was a medical student. In my third year of medical school, while perusing my voluminous 2- volume text on Internal Medicine, I came across the only two glossy pages with four pictures. I was instantly struck by a skin lesion that jumped off the page, drawing my attention to an identical lesion on my newlywed wife's back. The text below the photograph described a very aggressive and potentially fatal skin lesion: malignant melanoma.

I had not yet studied this cancer but quickly came up to speed. I was paralyzed with fear of the unknown as my wife and I were about to begin an incredibly dangerous and very possibly fatal journey. Fortunately, we were able to have the Melanoma fully resected with clear margins and disease-free lymph nodes. It was fortuitous that I stumbled across this cancer in its very early stage of growth, which allowed for a positive result.

Ten months later, prior to the start of my 4th year in medical school, my grandfather was diagnosed with gallbladder cancer, and he succumbed to the illness. I again encountered a cancer for which I had little knowledge nor practical experience. My family looked to me for guidance and comfort which I was not prepared to provide. I felt completely inadequate.

I did my internship and residency at the University of Utah and there I found many of the most prominent hematologists and oncologists in the country who had come to Salt Lake City to create a center of excellence in the study and treatment of cancer. I was exposed to much more cancer and leukemia than the average internal medicine program in the country. It was not unusual for me to be caring for more cancer patients than non-cancer patients. My education in medicine is grounded in those patients with acute leukemia, lung cancer, pancreatic cancer, lymphoma, and colon cancer.

However, it was my personal experience with seven Mohs surgeries for West Texas sun-exposed skin cancers, and my family's cancer battles that exposed me to the scope and challenges of the cancer journey. As members of my family battled cancer they continued to look to me for guidance and support. My siblings each had their own cancer journey. My sister was diagnosed with kidney cancer shortly following the loss of her father-in-law with his battle with colon cancer. She fortunately survived the cancer.

My younger brother, an award winning country music singer and writer, began his battle against cancer at the age of 40 when he was diagnosed with throat cancer, which has a 95% cure rate. After undergoing his initial successful treatment, his doctors recommended a laryngectomy to remove the remaining tissue in the damaged lining of the throat because recurrence of the cancer was inevitable. Because of his musical career my brother chose not to undergo the recommended surgery and 18 months later he passed following the recurrence of throat cancer.

During the past decade, I have been in the side car for both my son and wife in their struggles with cancer. My second son endured a horrific 5-year battle with appendix cancer before passing. The night before his celebration of life, I, and my wife, along with our extended family learned the awful news that she was diagnosed with metastatic adenocarcinoma. As I performed my son's service the next day, I knew my wife had terminal cancer and after a heroic 18-month battle, she too passed.

Most recently my dear childhood friend, Skitch, passed from the same rare form of cancer that took my son's life. Skitch was one of the 3 most influential men in my life. He gave me the courage and confidence to pursue my trajectory through a career in medicine and a side career in music. Helping his family with his celebration of life was devastating and rocked my soul.

I have sat at the bedside with two wives, my grandfather and grandmother, several dear friends and scores of patients as they passed taking their last breath. As a cancer treating physician, it is hard to put in words the sense of loss and devastation you experience when cancer takes a loved one or a patient.

Now with the understanding of my journey you see I view my provider role as a guide, an interpreter, and advocate for my patients, but I also am just another human spirit not unlike my patients. The difference is my work experience in medicine, underscored by my personal journey.

Hearing the words "you have cancer" changes one's life and you have just dropped a bomb on the patient and their family, and their lives will never be the same. My patients universally have a new understanding regarding the meaning of their life after hearing those words.

My provider role is to provide my medical knowledge with compassion, interpret various test results, explain treatment recommendations in understandable, non-medical terms, and provide an honest roadmap for their reluctant journey so the patient might develop realistic expectations and a perspective that will help ease the fear of the unknown. I begin the dialogue to help them acquire a new set of skills and tools to navigate the next chapter of their lives. As an advocate, I do all in my power to help provide safe passage throughout their cancer journey. I attempt to address all facets of their treatment, but there are several key items that need to be addressed as quickly as possible prior to embarking on their treatment.

The important items and concepts to address for the patient and their caregivers include:

the importance of hope, obtaining support, the importance of developing a meaningful life, and learning a new way to communicate with friends and family, including the most difficult conversation of all - saying goodbye. These key concepts are based on a foundation of the most accurate information including prognosis and a treatment plan in order to create real expectations for the impending future.

HOPE

Hope refers to simple expectations of outcomes and directly associated with quality of life.

Hope in broad terms rests on a foundation of truthful realistic expectations that consider the outcomes of different types of treatment.

The first goal is to begin building hope by providing a realistic roadmap that eliminates the patient's fear of the unknown. To achieve this result, I must provide honest answers to questions regarding the impact of the cancer and the treatment on a realistic prognosis, an honest prediction of the quality of life associated with the proposed treatment plan. I want patients and their families to understand "hope" takes on many faces and will be constantly changing as one moves through treatment regardless of the stage or outcome of treatment.

Initially, we might hope for complete eradication of the tumor, but later we are hopeful the chemotherapy infusion/treatment comes without obvious adverse reactions. When speaking about Hope, there are two important factors to consider:

First, I do not want patients to speculate about what is going to happen to them. A lack of factual data increases patients' fear and I want to be as accurate as possible and provide the patient a realistic view about future outcomes. Second, I want the patient to have the highest quality of life, even if their prognosis is not good and a negative outcome is likely.

It is difficult to discuss a cure for this awful disease. Hope cannot be based on the outcome.
Even if the disease is in remission, there is anxiety that the cancer will return and how long it will be before it does.

It is well established that a patient's positive attitude aids in recovery. The recovery healing factor is driven by the patient's positive attitude that helps to boost the immune system thus providing protection from infection and enhanced improvement in wound healing and repair. There are a variety of tools and skills that can be taught to the patient to aid in creating a positive attitude and help alleviate feelings of anxiety. At some cancer centers, like the Huntsman Cancer Center, programs are offered that help the patients learn concepts like mindfulness visualization techniques, yoga, massage, and meditation to help achieve a calm, peaceful mindset that help in the recovery process.

When patients ask about statistics and their prognosis, I speak in very generalized terms. I tell my patients that in the reported statistics and our experience their cancer was never part of the studies. I tell them they are bringing their own unique cancer, residing in their own unique body, with their own immune system, their level of conditioning, and their mental frame of mindset.

While their cancer is similar to others, it has never been treated with the drugs and modalities that we are preparing to use. Statistics are only rough guidelines, and it is difficult to extrapolate. I have seen many cancers that break the rules of large clinical studies. There are always outliers, and my patient might as well be one of those that have an unexpectedly good outcome.

Even with terminal cancer, there are many faces to hope. It is critical you do not pull the rug of Hope out from under the patient.

SUPPORT

There are many issues that require attention in the treatment of cancer. Very few people are completely knowledgeable of these issues or prepared to address them when they arise during a patient's cancer journey. A key area that every patient must confront is that of support and I am consistently amazed by the complexity and unpredictability of the needed support for the cancer traveler.

Each patient who is diagnosed with cancer is unique and will require different levels of support. They will present with their own specific cancer, at a specific stage of progression, and with a specific Kubler-Ross stage in the grief cycle (denial, anger, bargaining, depression, and acceptance), Some patients will start their journey with a broad range of family, friends, and community support, availability of caregivers, and with different financial capabilities. Others will have less comprehensive support networks.

A patient's geographic location also influences the availability of support for their journey. They may reside in an urban or in a rural setting. In an urban setting, the patient can live in the same city where they are 15 minutes from their treatment center. A cancer patient who lives in a community located hundreds of miles away from their medical provider or treatment center may require hours of travel and overnight lodging to receive the necessary treatment for their cancer without the support, comfort and familiarity of their home and community.

As other writers have noted, it is critically important to establish a strong, experienced support team as soon as possible. Support can be found in a variety of locations: at a dedicated cancer treatment organization, or from within the community, with an oncologist who is familiar with the treatment protocols for the patient's cancer, using a case manager from a home health service, and other community resources including patients who have experienced the same type of cancer, with your friends and family.

I have had the privilege of working within an integrated support system offering a comprehensive array of services for the patient and their caregiver(s).

There are numerous types of support available for the patient and their caregivers:

-A support team comprised of family, friends, and classmates, to help deal with the daily requirements of cancer treatment, including nutritional needs, help with the daily chores at home, transportation back and forth, and companionship.

-A multidisciplinary support team associated with your cancer-treating facility. The team will be multidisciplinary and with the ability to address all components of treatment involving:

Case Management, Social Work, Nursing needs, Home Health, Dietary, Physical Therapy, Legal Counselors help draft legal documents that reflect your end-of-life choices and wishes.

And Financial counselors helping to acquire financial aid and disability financial assistance, Spiritual support, and a Patient and Caregiver Library, specifically providing educational material and services offered for the patient and the caregivers.

You will be surprised how important and how often you will need these services.

-Online resources:
There are several incredibly informative online resources available to explain in lay terms details concerning your specific cancer type generalized options for treatment and outcomes.

Examples include the Mayo Clinic, MD Anderson, Sloan Kettering, the Huntsman Cancer Institute, Moffitt Cancer Center, and the American Cancer Society.

-Formal Organizations available include
Organizations found at your hospital, dedicated cancer centers, local community, state and national organizations, i.e., the National Cancer Society.

Warning:

I strongly caution patients to avoid non-accredited sites that can give you misinformation and non-standard-of-care treatment that can be so harmful. If one comes across one of these sites, I recommend they bring that information to their treating team for vetting to avoid potential harm.

There are multiple sites and well-wishers that will offer herbs, supplements, and non-conventual forms of treatments that could interfere with prescribed treatments or cause adverse reactions.

SAYING GOOD-BYE

My career choices over the duration of my career as a physician have primarily involved caring for critically ill patients who would either survive or pass. The need to effectively communicate with the patient, the family, and the care team members has been a constant over the years.

Providing quality care my for patients requires that I know the art and skill of effective communication, which I believe is one of the most important skills I have acquired during my medical career. Many people are uncomfortable communicating or just being present with the cancer patient, so acquiring better communication skills makes these interactions more comfortable for the patient, their caregivers and for me as the medical professional.

Communication becomes the constant in cancer treatment for everyone involved from the initial diagnosis until the final stage when it is necessary to say goodbye when a patient's condition reaches the point where they will not survive.

Over the many years of my career, I have established an approach to effective communication in the stage of saying goodbye. The first and possibly the most challenging skill is to develop an awareness that, at any given moment, every patient will be at a different stage of treatment and experiencing a wide range of emotions. With that understanding, there are several simple phrases and simple ways of being present that can help to achieve the goal of effective communication.

The goal is to create a positive, calming, comforting and informative atmosphere.

There are many ways to be present:
Being present - be there and be open to not talking or conversely talking very deeply.

Use simple phrases in the conversation with the patient.

Understand each person is different in the speed of coming to grips with their diagnosis - there are simply different paces and different understanding Sitting quietly with a loved one.

Do not treat the patient like they are different, treat them as the people they are.

Examples of important phrases in conversations with the patient:
This must be a tough time for you. I cannot imagine how you feel.
I am sorry you are going through something like this.
I do not know what to say.
I am here for you if you want to talk, or I am here for you just to be present.
How can I help you?
Do you want a ride to your appointment?
Would you like me to drop off some dinner?
I know staying positive is hard?
There are key questions we should ask the patient while we are with them:
How are you really feeling?
How can I best support your needs?
Ask for feedback on their course of treatment. What can we do differently or better?
We must remember the power of words and how we communicate with anyone that is healing.

Saying Goodbye

Saying goodbye is the hardest thing that any of us do in caring for patients. At some point, saying goodbye is a conversation the provider, staff, patient, family and friends, and other caregivers must undertake. One should say goodbye early and often. Do not delay. Things happen with a speed and consequences that cannot be anticipated.

From my personal experience saying goodbye to my sweet wife and soulmate, Liz, the opportunity to say goodbye was almost completely lost. She unexpectedly developed a state of confusion lasting many weeks prior to her passing. I thought I had missed the opportunity to share our last words and goodbye and I was so incredibly sad.

Liz's confusion interfered in the ability to effectively communicate, and the course of events almost cost us the opportunity to say goodbye. Fortunately, several days before she passed the confusion cleared for 36 hours. She wanted to speak individually to me and each one of our children. Her conversation and message were so sweet and loving yet so incredibly powerful and impactful. She left each one of us with a personalized message.

In the end, Liz was the one who was so compassionate yet strong and fearless. She was so grateful to have had such a loving caring family. She expressed her love and gratitude just as we also did.

The thought of possibly missing that goodbye is unbearable.
I will leave this section with this advice.

When saying goodbye, use the time to express your love and appreciation for each other. Express your love early and often.

Be reassuring and honest, and it is so important to be grateful because time will eventually come to an end.

Living A Meaningful Life

"Quality of life" is a recurring theme in most cancer treatment literature. Quality of life or the promise of a quality of life is the main goal and reason to pursue cancer treatment. For the patient and provider, the absence of a quality of life becomes a hard stop in pursuing cancer treatment.

Regardless of whether the cancer is terminal or not, I tell my patients that the cancer gives us many things and one of them is what I consider an incredibly special gift. That gift is we are reminded of our own mortality and that we all have a limited time to live on this earth which will come to an end one day. Cancer brings that reality into sharp focus.

The reason I consider this to be a special gift resides in the fact most people do not live a life that acknowledges the transient nature of our lives. My cancer patients have no choice but to come face to face with their own mortality and the meaning of life.

I advise the patient to not stop living and remind them that our purpose and what we do defines living a life with meaning. I then ask the patient what would a meaningful life look like to them?

When an answer is given, some will affirm a purpose and living a meaningful life, but many come up blank. I then suggest to both the patient and their caregivers an additional purpose to consider for their remaining time, however long that might be. I suggest they consider a life of service to others in whatever capacity they are capable.

Providing a service to others would surely be meaningful and it could be as simple as sitting with a fellow patient during a chemotherapy infusion, working in a soup kitchen, reading to a fellow soul residing in a nursing home or working at any facility that serves people in need. I promise them that participating in the purpose of helping our fellow man will bring a meaningfulness to their life that they may never have experienced. I tell them service to others will become an important aid in their cancer treatment. It will give them a meaningful life.

Final Thoughts

I am a Liver Transplant physician, and it is difficult to put into words the feelings that washed over me as I have struggled drafting these words as it has forced me to revisit so many memories. It truly has been like pulling a scab off a healing wound. This introspection has been so important and valuable, though incredibly difficult. As you have read, I approach cancer carrying a unique lifetime story of formal education and personal experience.

Cancer has been a constant in my career as a physician and my adult life. I am a physician that treats patients with cancer. I have dealt with cancer as a father, a brother, a grandson, a husband, and a friend. Finally, I am a cancer survivor. As a health care provider, I have traveled with them as they undertook the reluctant, incredibly difficult cancer journey. As a physician, I have been blessed with the opportunity to participate in the care of this incredibly special group of patients.

Notes From The Field

Hospice and Palliative Care

By
Stacey Akeley, R.N., B.S.N.

The five themes expressed in this book, Being a Cancer Patient, Obtaining Support, Hope, Saying Goodbye, and Living a Meaningful Life, embrace the meaning and goals of Hospice and Palliative Care. Palliative care, as defined by the Center to Advance Palliative Care (CAPC), is specialized medical care for people living with a serious illness. This type of care is focused on providing relief from the symptoms and stress of a serious illness. The goal is to improve the quality of life for both the patient and the family.

Palliative care is provided by a specially- trained team of palliative care physicians, nurses, and other specialists who work together with the patient's other doctors to provide an extra layer of support. It is appropriate at any age and at any stage in a serious illness, and it can be provided along with curative treatment.

Hospice is an insurance benefit offered by Medicare and some insurances. The benefit offers Palliative Care for a person with a terminal illness whose doctor believes he or she has six months or less to live if the illness runs its natural course.

Hospice and Palliative care focus on providing comprehensive care and comfort for the patient and their family, but, in hospice, medical treatments focus on comfort rather than cure. The hospice benefit includes 24/7 on-call nursing support and regular visits, a full team of specially trained volunteers, chaplains, social workers, hospice aides, nurses, and physicians, working together and along with the patient's current physician. Nurses provide highly skilled care and support to maximize comfort and minimize pain and other symptoms.

Hospice aides assist with personal care needs. Volunteers offer non-medical aid and support and are an essential part of the hospice team. Social workers provide counseling and support about what to expect. Chaplains offer spiritual care and support. Bereavement counselors are available to help caregivers with anticipatory grief and ongoing support up to 13 months after the death of their loved one.

Many people are afraid of hospice, not understanding the many benefits it provides, and enter hospice with only days to weeks left to live. As my hospice agency states, "Hospice doesn't mean you're giving up, it means you're taking charge". The hospice team helps patients and caregivers understand what Being a Cancer Patient means to them by exploring, through skillful conversations, what matters to them. They help patients understand, reflect, and discuss goals for future care and make decisions in the context of their values and beliefs. The team offers Support by exploring worries, hopes, and goals and clarifying what is most important.

The hospice team helps patients look at Hope in this way: hope for the best, attend to the present, and prepare for the worst. The spiritual care provided by the chaplains, social workers, volunteers, and bereavement counselors explore stages of grief and help patients and caregivers with Saying Goodbye. The team looks at care of patients and families at end of life as not dying of cancer but living as fully and comfortably and as aligned with their wishes and goals as possible and therefore Living a Meaningful Life to the very end.

Important References/Resources include:
Center to Advance Palliative Care (CAPC) An organization dedicated to increasing the availability of quality, equitable health care for people living with a serious illness; provides health care providers with training, tools, and technical assistance to meet this need.

GetPalliativeCare.org For patients and families to learn about palliative care and access the national Palliative Care Provider Directory Medicare.gov To learn more about the hospice benefit National Hospice and Palliative Care Organization (NHPCO) An organization for providers and professionals who care for people with serious and life-limiting illnesses

EPILOGUE

Those Three Words

By
David W. Persky, Ph.D., J.D.

"You have cancer." Three terrifying words for a cancer patient and for the patient's cancer caregiver(s). They are also difficult words for the medical professionals who deal with cancer and work with cancer patients at various stages along the cancer journey.

Our writers have provided us with us some insights of their careers and how they came to treat patients with cancer. Kevin and Lawrence grew up in medical families, but they took different paths to their medical careers. Kevin aspired to be a urologist like his father and attended medical school at St. George's University after earning his BS Biology at the University of South Carolina. He then completed a residency program in surgery in New York and a urology residency program at the University of South Florida. Lawrence grew up wanting to be a doctor but explored other careers and earned a Ph.D. in Chemistry at Yale and briefly had a career outside of health care before deciding to earn for his medical degree at the University of Pittsburgh. He did a residency at the University of Pennsylvania and briefly considered a career in ophthalmology before finding his passion in radiation oncology. Helen wanted to be a doctor as a young girl and earned a degree in English. She worked for a pediatric hematologist in Boston which reignited her interest in a career in medicine. Helen returned to earn her medical degree at Tufts University as an "older" student when she was 27 and found her passion in oncology. Elliot earned his undergraduate degree in Cell Biology at UConn and a graduate degree in Human Physiology at Georgetown before matriculating at the University of Maryland for his medical degree and a residency in OB/Gyn. Stacy earned her RN certificate and a BSN and spent a significant portion of her career as a Certified Hospice and Palliative Care Nurse. Ray Thomason earned his undergraduate degree at SMU in Biology and his MD at the University of Texas Southwestern Medical School before his internship and residency in Gastroenterology at the University of Utah.

Our medical professionals initially found themselves uncertain about exactly how to treat the various cancers their patients presented while under their care, but over time learned and developed their own protocols for the cancer cases they treated. Ray's exposure to cancer came when he was a medical student and noticed a picture of a melanoma in a textbook that looked remarkably like the lesion on his wife's back. He was not prepared to learn about cancer but found himself put into that position to help ensure that his wife's melanoma did not metastasize. He later learned about other cancers as members of his family experienced cancer and looked to him for help.

As noted by our writers, each patient's journey is different. Our writers thoroughly review the patient's medical records and seek the best course of treatment to help their patients while trying to respect the patients' needs and wishes. The fundamental question asked is: "How can I best help the patient in this journey?"

The best strategies to provide optimum care and help for cancer traveler are not always evident at the outset of the journey. It takes time to determine what will work best for the patient in his/her situation. What works for one cancer patient does not necessarily work for another in the same way. Our medical providers have shown that it takes time to discern the appropriate approach for each patient who is dealing with the most difficult health struggle of their lives. It is an "uncomfortable reality" for everyone involved in the cancer journey. As all cancer travelers, caregivers and medical professionals have learned, life is not fair, and it is not an easy process.

One concept that is a concern for each of our writers was that of time. It is the great unknown that comes with the cancer diagnosis. The obvious first step taken by each of the medical professionals is to spend time learning as much as they can about the type of cancer presented by the patient. In some cases, the treatment options are clear after thoroughly reading the patient's charts and having the initial consultation with the patient and, in many cases, the patient's spouse or significant other. In other cases, treatment options are not readily evident.

There is a consistent pattern in the individual approaches followed by our writers. They want to make sure they communicate clearly with their patients so there is no confusion about the course of treatment and the desired outcome for the patient and the patient's support network. Each of our medical professionals spends time with exam to help him develop the individual course of treatment that is most appropriate for them. This is essential to help each patient achieve a sense of meaning their life and a legacy to leave behind if their prognosis is not good.

Our writers each strive to be a resource for their patients. They do not provide insight on how to live a meaningful life, but they can help them find support groups that are available for the patients' specific type of cancer. The importance of good support networks for the patient is stressed by each of our writers. Some patients quickly locate programs in their communities to provide needed (and sometimes necessary) support for them and for their significant others. While support may be evident to some patients who readily seek others who are on a similar journey, others may be reluctant to seek support and our writers each strive to emphasize the benefits of support during and after the patient's treatment for their cancer. Ray goes a bit further and cautions his patients about questionable online resources that may offer a "cure" for cancer but are in actuality scams to get money without providing a cure or any meaningful support.

Another aspect of time for the medical professional is preparing for the end if the cancer patient's condition is terminal. It is not easy for the medical provider, and each has established a practice that strives to maintain the patient's quality of life and to allow them to die with dignity. They cannot tell the patient what to say or how to feel, but they want to focus on the positives for the patient and the patient's support network. Elliot wants his patients to have no regrets at the end and to "clear the air" and dwell on the positives of their lives. Helen has learned throughout her practice that is beneficial to allow the patient to spend their remaining time the way they choose. They can choose where they will say their good-byes. Some patients will stay in the hospital and others will decide to return home or to hospice for their final days. Hospice programs like Stacey's provide a wonderful service to the patients and their families and ensure the patient is in a good place and comfortable, surrounded by their loved ones. Our writers each want the patient to take whatever time is needed to share their thoughts and emotions and to reflect on the positives of their life.

We know our medical professionals have remarkably busy schedules and have had to balance their schedules and their limited freedom to share their insights for this book and we thank them for their time and contributions to this project.
David Persky, Ph.D., J.D.

Got an idea for a book? Contact Curry Brothers Publishing, LLC. We are not satisfied until your publishing dreams come true. We specialize in all genres of books, especially religion, self-help, leadership, family history, poetry, and children's literature. There is an African Proverb that confirms, *"When an elder dies, a library closes."* Be careful who tells your family history. Our staff will navigate you through the entire publishing process, and we take pride in going the extra mile in meeting your publishing goals. Improving the world one book at a time!

Curry Brothers Publishing, LLC PO Box 247 Haymarket, VA 20168 (719) 466-7518 & (615) 347-9124

Visit us at: http://www.currybrotherspublishing.com

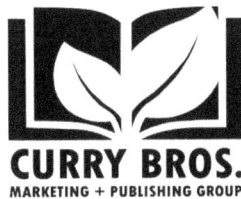

CURRY BROS.
MARKETING + PUBLISHING GROUP

9 798987 362341